The Pregnancy BOOK

by Doctors & Staff of

THE ROYAL HOSPITAL FOR WOMEN

A BAY BOOKS PUBLICATION
An imprint of HarperCollinsPublishers

First published in Australia in 1982 by Bay Books
Reprinted in 1987, 1992
This edition completely revised and updated in 1993 by Bay Books, of

CollinsAngus&Robertson Publishers Pty Limited (ACN 009 913 517)
A division of HarperCollinsPublishers (Australia) Pty Limited
25 Ryde Road, Pymble NSW 2073, Australia

HarperCollinsPublishers (New Zealand) Limited
31 View Road, Glenfield, Auckland 10, New Zealand

HarperCollinsPublishers Limited
77-85 Fulham Palace Road, London W6 8JB, United Kingdom

National Library of Australia
Cataloguing-in-Publication data:

Completely rev. ed.
Includes index.

ISBN 1 86378 026 2.

1. Pregnancy. 2. Childbirth. I. Royal Hospital for Women
(Paddington, NSW)

612.63

Printed in Singapore

8 7 6 5 4
97 96 95 94 93

CONTRIBUTORS

The contributors to the original edition of this book (published in 1982) were all members of the staff of the Royal Hospital for Women, Sydney, at time of original publication.

The following people contributed to the original edition of this book:

Mark Beale, MB, BS, FRCOG, FRACOG, Obstetrician and Gynaecologist

Michael Bennett, MD, ChB (UCT), FCOG (SA), FRCOG, FRACOG, DDU

Christine Borthwick, BSc, Dip Nutrition and Dietetics, Dietician

Christopher Bradbury, MB, BS, MRCOG, FRACOG, Obstetrician and Gynaecologist

Ann Burleigh, RGN, RMN, Postnatal Ward Charge Sister

Howard Chilton, MB, BS, LRCP, MRCS, MRCP, DCH, Director of Newborn Services

Dick Climie, MB, ChB, FFARCS, FFARACS, Director of Anaesthesia

Ian Cope, MD, BS, FCRCS, FRACS, FRCOG, FRACOG, Obstetrician and Gynaecologist

Geraldine Dolin, SRN, SCM, Nursing Sister

Mary Field, BSoc Stud, Senior Social Worker

C.C. Fisher, MB, BS, FRCOG, FRACGP, FRACOG, Director of Fetal Intensive Care

Patricia Fleming, Dip Physio (Qld), MAPA, Chief Physiotherapist

William Garrett, MD, BS, DPhil (Oxon), FRACS, FRCSEd, FRCOG, FRACOG, FRACR (Hon), Director of Diagnostic Ultrasound

Stephen P. Gatt, MD, LRCP, MRCS, FRARACS, FFA Intensive Care

Judy Gray, RN, RM, Midwife

John Greenwell, MB, BS, FRCOG, FRACMA, FRACOG, General Medical Superintendent

Mary Hancock, SNR, SCM, Nursing Sister

Grahame Harris, MB, BS, FRCOG, FRACOG, Obstetrician and Gynaecologist

Michael Harris, MB, BS, DCH (RPC&S), FRCP (Lond), FRACP, Paediatrician

Marie Hiscock, RGN, RMN, RM'craft, Assistant Matron

Yvonne Holcombe, MB, BS, FRCPA, Pathologist

Trevor Johnson, MB, BS, MRCOG, FRACOG, Obstetrician and Gynaecologist

Bruce Kendall, MB, BS, DGO (Syd), FRACOG, Obstetrician and Gynaecologist

Stephen Kovacs, MB, BS, MRCOG, FRACOG, Obstetrician and Gynaecologist

Christine Marr, BSc, Dip Nutrition and Dietetics, Dietician

Bettie Michie, SNR, SCM, ADNE (Cumberland), Nursing Sister

Margaret Sheens, RCN, RMN, RM'craft, RPN, Community Liaison Sister

Stephen Steigrad, MB, BS, FRCSEd, FRACOG, FRCOG, Deputy General Medical Superintendent

Jill Talty, BSoc.Wk., Senior Social Worker

Peter Warren, MB, ChB, Dip Obst MRACR, Staff Specialist in Diagnostic Ultrasound

Debbie Wass, MRCOG, FRACOG, Lecturer UNSW

The following people (who are members of the staff of the Royal Hospital for Women) revised and updated this edition:

Michael Bennett, MD, ChB (UCT), FCOG (SA), FRCOG, FRACOG, DDU; Professor of Obstetrics and Gynaecology, UNSW and Head of the School of Obstetrics and Gynaecology; Director of Obstetrics and Gynaecology, Royal Hospital for Women

Christopher Bradbury, MB, BS, MRCOG, FRACOG, Obstetrician and Gynaecologist

Howard Chilton, MB, BS, LRCP, MRCS, MRCP, DCH, Director of Newborn Services

C.C. Fisher, MB, BS, FRCOG, FRACGP, FRACOG, Director of Fetal Intensive Care

Joy Heads, Lactation Consultant

We acknowledge with gratitude the assistance of Helen Damdo, Helen Jarman, Glynn McNally and Peter Warren for making it possible to take photographs at the hospital; and Glynn McNally for supplying ultrasound images.

Our thanks to HJ Heinz Co. Aust. Ltd for supplying some photographs for this book.

FOREWORD TO THE THIRD EDITION

It is ten years since The *Pregnancy Book* was first published. This is a new and third edition. This fact alone speaks volumes for the original gap in information that this book filled for so many women. It recognises clearly the continuing demand for this type of information about all aspects of pregnancy, good and bad. This information is more readily available in this book than in any other.

The moving spirit behind the first two editions was the late Bruce Kendall, a much loved and respected senior obstetrician at the Royal Women's Hospital in Paddington. Professor Michael Bennett, Drs Christopher Bradbury, Howard Chilton and Col Fisher are to be congratulated for what will inevitably prove to be a very popular third edition.

As I did ten years ago, I warmly commend this book. I now know it will reach the wide audience it deserves.

RODNEY P. SHEARMAN, AO

Rodney P. Shearman, MD (Syd), DGO (Syd), FRCOG, PRACOG, Professor of Obstetrics and Gynaecology, University of Sydney. Head, Division of Obstetrics and Gynaecology, Royal Prince Alfred Hospital.

Former President, The Royal Australian College of Obstetricians and Gynaecologists.

CONTENTS

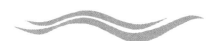

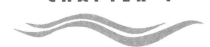

CHAPTER 1

LET'S HAVE A BABY

Preparation for Pregnancy

Pregnancy has both physical and emotional aspects which must be faced over the nine months. Many of these aspects produce very pleasant sensations and rewarding emotional responses, and many of them do not.

The physical and emotional problems which emerge both during and after pregnancy may make couples feel unable to cope with what others regard as a normal process. This feeling of inadequacy is very common during pregnancy, in labour and in the weeks after delivery and in most cases it is completely unwarranted. In such a mood, the slightest departure from what the mother and father-to-be see as the normal course of events can indicate to them a state of near-disaster. The 'normal' course of events, however, varies from woman to woman and from pregnancy to pregnancy.

Pregnancy can be nice or nasty

▼▼▼

There may be anxiety about coping with pregnancy

▼▼▼

Friends and neighbours, sisters and parents may present a picture of their own pregnancy and labour and tend to assume that others will have the same experience. With this background of conflicting advice, the ability to listen and interpret becomes important. Pregnancy can be an exciting and happy time. There are increasing numbers of books, magazine articles, videos, TV shows and dependable professionals for a couple to be able to get the facts. The emotions may be new and different but having confidence in one's own good sense and allowing oneself to be a pregnant woman, rather than a woman who just happens to be pregnant, will help a lot. A pregnant woman is not an alien creature unable to function intelligently but she is allowed to be different and special.

MOTIVATION *for* PREGNANCY

People have babies for many different reasons. It may be that they did not use effective contraception; or that all their friends are pregnant; or that the timing seems right.

By the age of 18 some women may have formed a clear concept of the number of children they wish to have.

They may persist in trying to make the wish come true, even when reason tells them they should not. Other women wish to avoid pregnancy either completely or at least for a very long period after marriage. Some see pregnancy not only as a normal occurrence but often as the only reason for the relationship or the marriage, and there are certainly some men who think like this.

Men on the other hand may be a little confused by what is expected of them and they may simply go along with what their partners wish. However, they are becoming more involved these days in the decision whether to have children or not. Couples are now seeing child rearing as a shared responsibility and often arrangements are made whereby they both help out. Childcare centres are becoming increasingly competent and an excellent centre may in fact stimulate and enhance the welfare of the child.

It is now virtually universal that the male partner attends prenatal classes and is present at the birth. He is able to help, remind, comfort and console during pregnancy and the labour. Most women say that they could never have managed without their partner. Of course they could have, but it might not have been nearly as memorable nor as enjoyable. No man should feel coerced into attending the birth — it should be voluntary. In fact many men feel like stretching their legs and having something to eat during the birth process. Very few men faint and no one is compelled to look if they think it is a little messy or disturbing.

Many women conceive because they are sick of using contraceptives, particularly the Pill. Some deliberately stop taking the Pill because they fear it might cause them to become infertile. Others are not using contraceptives because they think they are sterile or have been told they may be infertile as a result of some pelvic infection. Many of these women wish to prove their fertility rather than produce a baby and may not have thought beyond the actual conception.

A few women try to use a pregnancy to force a marriage and some try to conceive in order to become a single parent, to have something of their own to love. Probably the biggest myth about pregnancy is that it will hold together a failing relationship or marriage. A pregnancy started for reasons that see the baby as an object or tool, rather than a person, may well create more problems than it solves.

Many pregnancies are motivated by both partners wanting to develop their relationship further, feeling that they are ready for the responsibilities of parenthood. Many theorists believe that couples come to a stage in their lives and relationships when instinctively they are ready to have a family. This readiness is similar to a child's readiness to walk, an adolescent's readiness to be interested in the opposite sex or a young person's readiness to leave home. The readiness for parenthood grows from the satisfaction the partners have in their relationship with each other and from their mutual desire to move forward.

PLANNING

With this level of motivation, the question of planning and timing will probably be considered. Preparation and planning both require one basic ingredient: communication between partners. Couples who have been together only a short time may not yet have established a good pattern of communication. Couples who have been together for a long time may have become so comfortable and intuitive in each other's company that they have partly lost the need and perhaps even the capacity to share with one another those personal and intimate thoughts, fears and feelings, which are part of facing an important change. Unless both partners are interested in and look forward to what is coming and can discuss it together, there are going to be many problems to solve.

For those couples with an unexpected pregnancy there may be particularly difficult times ahead. Each may feel some guilt: for example, that one partner has been placed in an economically difficult position or that the other has to cope with an unplanned pregnancy. Hard as it may be, sharing these fears and feelings is likely to help and not hinder the relationship, by creating a bond in planning together for the one thing in common: the expected baby.

Planning can, and indeed should, include a visit to a family doctor, preferably one who knows both partners. It provides an opportunity to identify and treat minor disorders that may be present, and to find the occasional major problem which might lead to serious consequences. It also allows for a discussion of anxieties about pregnancy and an explanation of many of the myths and old wives' tales that surround pregnancy and labour.

FERTILITY

Becoming pregnant can be easy — sometimes. However, it does not always happen straightaway and to understand why, it helps to know a little about fertility and how we reproduce.

Some 15 per cent of couples (1 in 7) are relatively or completely infertile. About one-third of these show no abnormality and will eventually conceive although it may take a year or more for them to do so. Of the remaining two-thirds the infertility problem is divided fairly evenly between those cases where the husband is infertile, where the wife is infertile and where infertility is shared between the two. Many of these infertility problems can now be solved by modern medicine and surgery.

A couple can be 'ready' to have a baby
▼▼▼

Communication is important
▼▼▼

Becoming pregnant isn't always easy
▼▼▼

The effect of even relative infertility on any couple will vary with their personalities and their eagerness to conceive and will range from quiet resignation to acute anxiety. Continued failure to conceive can lead to depression and crying spells at each menstrual period or to aggressive behaviour which can colour the whole personality and greatly disturb the relationship. The stress of modern living combined with anxiety about continued failure to conceive can itself cause a particular type of infertility.

When pregnancy does at last occur after a period of infertility, there is an immediate feeling of success in both partners but usually this is tempered by a degree of anxiety, which is greater than it need be, about the outcome of the pregnancy.

Anxiety can
cause
infertility
▼▼▼

PHYSIOLOGICAL PREPARATION *for* PREGNANCY

The childbearing period of a woman's life begins some time between the ages of 15 and 18 and finishes usually in the mid-40s. During this fertile phase of life the body prepares itself for a pregnancy each month by a complex interplay of hormones (chemical 'messengers') produced by the hypothalamus and pituitary gland at the base of the brain and by the ovaries in the pelvis. The hormones are carried by the bloodstream all over the body and seek out and interact with the organs which are receptive to them.

This hormonal activity begins well before the fertile phase, commencing several years before the onset of menstruation. It is responsible for the initial growth and development of the breasts and genital organs in the young girl and for the gradual changes in the body shape which precede the first period at about 11 or 12 years of age.

The initial stimulus for hormonal activity comes from the hypothalamus, a portion of the brain immediately above the pituitary gland. At first the stimulus is slow and steady, and leads to the production of a hormone from the pituitary which stimulates the ovary to produce the female hormones (oestrogens). The oestrogens promote the growth of the breasts and female genitals including the vagina, uterus and Fallopian tubes and more particularly the lining of the uterus which grows and thickens under the influence of the hormones.

After a while the hypothalamus begins to regulate the hormone production in a cyclical fashion. The cyclical fall in oestrogen production leads to a breakdown of the lining of the uterus (the endometrium). The shedding of this lining, together with some blood, constitutes the menstrual period.

The first few menstrual cycles are usually irregular and not associated with the release of an egg from the ovary. Some time between the ages of 15 and 18, the stimulus from the hypothalamus to the pituitary and thence to the ovary is intense enough to trigger a follicle to rupture through the surface of the ovary and release an egg cell (ovum). This event, called ovulation, is usually associated with regular menstrual periods. It occurs approximately every 28 days, 14 days before the onset of a period.

Following ovulation the follicle from which the egg came is stimulated by a second pituitary hormone to develop into a corpus luteum. This is a yellow organ which grows in the ovary and produces the second ovarian hormone, progesterone, as well as smaller amounts of oestrogen. The two hormones, oestrogen and progesterone, build up and thicken the lining of the uterus in preparation for the entry of the fertilised egg into the uterus.

Should the egg fail to be fertilised, the corpus luteum continues to function for a further 10 to 12 days before rather suddenly ceasing to produce hormones. This sudden drop in circulating oestrogen and progesterone causes the lining to break down, hence menstruation begins, and the whole cycle is ready to be repeated.

Hormones regulate reproduction in men and women.

Similar hormone activity occurs in the young boy, but here the stimulus from the hypothalamus to the pituitary gland continues in a steady fashion all his life and no cycle can be recognised. The pituitary hormone stimulates the testicles to produce testosterone, the hormone which causes the usual changes associated with puberty. Eventually it also stimulates the production of adult sperm cells, many millions of which are ejaculated by the male at each sexual act.

Once in the vagina, these sperm cells travel with a swimming movement into the uterus and out along the Fallopian tubes. If they are deposited in the vagina either a few days before or at the time of ovulation, they meet the egg cell which has been released at ovulation and which is now in the outer part of the Fallopian tube. One of the sperm cells unites with the egg cell, and they fuse in a process called fertilisation. The fertilised egg receives half of its genetic material from the female and half from the male, and now contains in a single cell considerably smaller than the head of a pin, all the potential for a unique new human.

Ovulation is the release of an egg and occurs 14 days before a period

▼▼▼

The menstrual cycle

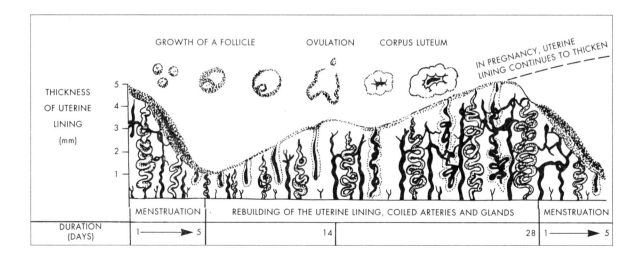

Once fertilisation occurs, the fertilised egg cell begins dividing as it moves down the Fallopian tube towards the uterus. Within four to five days it has increased in size several times, and about seven days following ovulation it implants itself in the prepared lining of the uterus. The outer cells of the embryo produce a pituitary-like hormone which prevents menstruation from occurring. The embryo embeds itself deeply into the thick lining of the uterus where a rich source of food and oxygen is available for its further growth and development.

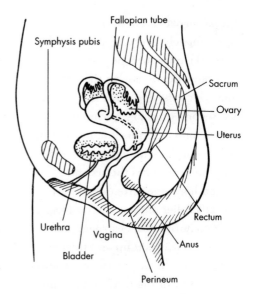

Female urogenital organs

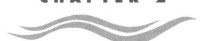

CHAPTER 2

HOW DOES OUR BABY GROW?

Growth of the embryo and fetus

We apologise for the complexity of parts of this chapter which may be hard to follow without some elementary knowledge of human biology. Unfortunately much of the early development of the embryo can only be seen under a microscope. It is hoped that the illustrations will help in understanding this section.

All human life, and indeed all life on earth, is centred in the structure of cells and their capacity to divide and reproduce themselves. Without this capacity we would never recover from the many cuts, abrasions and fractures that occur during a lifetime.

Most of the cells in our bodies are adult or mature cells and when

> *We are all made up of millions of cells*
>
> ▼▼▼

these divide and multiply they reproduce identical images of themselves, be they skin or bone or muscle cells or more complicated cells such as those in the internal organs. Some of our cells are immature cells, like the primitive cells in the bone marrow, which are capable of dividing and developing into any of the cellular structures in the blood, such as red blood cells or the several varieties of white blood cells. Others, such as many of the cells in the brain, are so highly specialised and mature, that they are incapable of dividing and multiplying and when destroyed by injury or disease, are lost forever.

CHROMOSOMES and GENES

The capacity of any cell to divide is centred in the nucleus of the cell. When the nucleus is viewed under a high-powered microscope, it is seen to be composed of a series of interwoven structures made up of complex chains of protein molecules. These structures are called chromosomes.

Each species of plant and animal life has a distinctive number of chromosomes in each cell nucleus. Man, the most complex of all species on earth, has 46 chromosomes, arranged in 23 pairs in the nucleus of every cell in his body. Each chromosome has a characteristic shape and size, but in all of them the chain of protein molecules is arranged in the same double spiral, like two interwoven springs, called a double helix.

Within each chromosome are small protein groupings known as genes and the number of genes making up each chromosome is very large. A conservative estimate of the number of genes in the 46 chromosomes would be well over 100 000.

SEX CHROMOSOMES

Twenty-two of the 23 pairs of chromosomes in each cell are the same in males and females and are known as autosomes. One pair, the sex chromosomes, is different. In females it consists of two X chromosomes, so named because of their shape. In males it consists of an X and a Y chromosome.

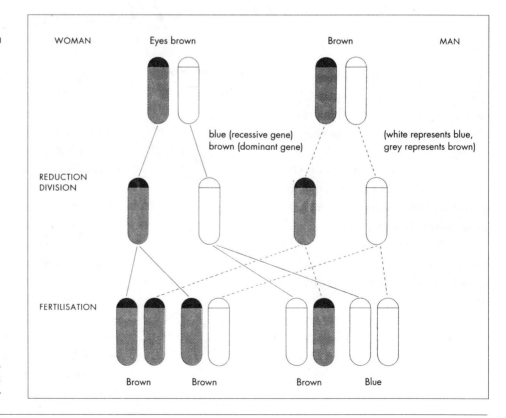

WOMAN   Eyes brown   Brown   MAN

blue (recessive gene)
brown (dominant gene)

(white represents blue,
grey represents brown)

REDUCTION
DIVISION

FERTILISATION

Brown   Brown   Brown   Blue

*Genetic
transmission
of eye colour*

CELL DIVISION *and* GROWTH

When an ordinary cell divides, a process known as mitosis, each of the paired chromosomes lays down alongside itself an exact copy, completely duplicating all its genes. When the cell divides, each doubled chromosome splits down the middle, one half going to each of the daughter cells. The daughter cells become complete copies of the original parent cell with the original genetic coding which is totally characteristic of that individual.

REDUCTION DIVISION

However, in the sex glands, the ovary and the testes, a special kind of cell division, called a reduction division (meiosis), occurs during the development of the ovum and the sperm. In this division the chromosome pairs separate bodily so that the resulting cells receive only one member of each pair, and thus contain only 23 single chromosomes.

When an egg is fertilised by a sperm, each chromosome in the nucleus of the sperm pairs up with its corresponding partner in the nucleus of the egg. The fertilised egg then contains all the potential for a new individual with 46 chromosomes arranged in 23 pairs, half from the father and half from the mother. All subsequent growth of this cell then occurs by ordinary division (mitosis).

Many of the physical characteristics of this new individual will be determined by the mix of the genes contributed by the two parents.

Some genes are dominant: they produce their characteristic effects even when only one of the paired chromosomes carries this gene. Other genes are recessive: both of the paired chromosomes have to carry the same gene to produce the genetic effect.

So, two brown-eyed individuals carrying the dominant gene for brown eyes on one chromosome and the recessive gene for blue eyes on the other will have the potential for producing a blue-eyed child in the ratio of one to three.

SEX DETERMINATION

As already explained, each egg and sperm contain only half of the adult number of chromosomes; they therefore each contain 22 autosomes and one sex chromosome. Hence, all egg cells contain 22 + X chromosomes, and sperms contain 22 + X or 22 + Y chromosomes, in equal numbers.

If an egg is fertilised by a sperm containing 22 + X chromosomes, the total number of chromosomes in each cell of the embryo will be 44 + X + X and the result will be a female child. However, should the sperm contain 22 + Y chromosomes, a male child will result.

This would suggest that equal numbers of male and female children should be conceived. In fact, more males are conceived than females in the ratio of 105:100. One explanation offered for this is that the small size of the Y chromosome allows those sperm carrying the Y to reach the egg cell well ahead of the slower X-

Normal cell division
▼▼▼

Reduction division
▼▼▼

Female is XX, male is XY
▼▼▼

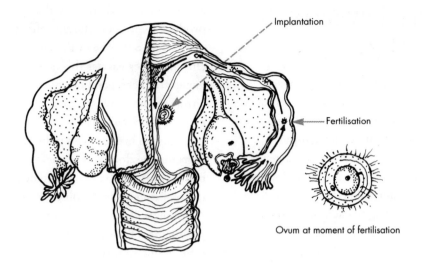

Implantation

Fertilisation

Ovum at moment of fertilisation

carrying sperms. This explanation is probably too simple but it has prompted the theory that there is a greater chance of producing a male baby by a single act of intercourse immediately before ovulation occurs. However, another explanation for the male-female ratio could also be the fact that X-carrying sperms do not live as long as Y-carrying sperms.

DIVISION *of the* FERTILISED EGG

Fertilisation occurs when one sperm penetrates the lining membrane of the egg cell. The chromosomes separate from the nuclei of the sperm and egg cell and fuse together to form a single nucleus with the adult number of chromosomes. The single cell then divides into two cells, which in turn divide to produce four cells, each of which then divides producing eight cells, and embryonic development is underway. So with each cell division, occurring about every 12 hours, the number of cells doubles from two to four to eight to 16 to 32 and so on.

Fertilisation is thought to occur when the egg is in the outer part of the Fallopian tube. The fertilised ovum is moved slowly along the tube by waves of muscular activity in the wall of the tube and by the flicking action of tiny 'hairs' (cilia) on the cells lining the tube. The fertilised ovum reaches the uterus in four to five days by which time it will consist of 32 or more cells still encased in the original smooth membrane of the egg.

IMPLANTATION

Soon after reaching the uterus, a cavity forms in the mass of cells, and the outer membrane disintegrates. This allows the sticky outer cells to attach to the wall of the uterus and become incorporated into it. This occurs about seven days after fertilisation and sometimes produces a small amount of bleeding known as implantation bleeding. As this bleeding occurs one week before a menstrual period is expected, it is often mistaken for a normal but early period, and this can cause confusion later when estimating the date of arrival of the baby.

The fertilised ovum with its cavity, looking somewhat like a diamond ring, is now called the blastocyst. It embeds with the nubble of cells (the 'diamond' of the 'ring') most deeply embedded. This nubble of cells is called the inner cell mass and from it will develop the embryo.

The outer layer of cells which are invading the lining of the uterus are called the trophoblastic cells and are concerned with the nutrition of the embryo. They grow very rapidly at this stage, developing into the placenta and the outermost membrane, the chorion (see below).

The inner cell mass assumes a flattened disc shape (the embryonic disc) with a separate sheet of cells either side, ectoderm above and endoderm below. From the edge of the ectodermal surface a layer of cells (the amnion) grows to form a fluid-filled cavity (the amniotic cavity), while the undersurface of the embryonic disc (the endoderm) lines the blastocystic cavity which is now called the yolk sac.

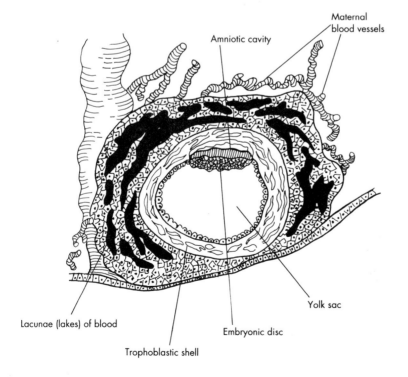

Maternal blood vessels

Amniotic cavity

Lacunae (lakes) of blood

Trophoblastic shell

Embryonic disc

Yolk sac

Diagram of a human implantation at 12 days

The food supply must be established first

▼▼▼

The amniotic cavity protects the growing embryo

▼▼▼

The source of the food supply is now centred in the placenta

▼▼▼

GROWTH *of the* PLACENTA *and* MEMBRANES

Meanwhile the outer trophoblastic cells have grown into the lining of the uterus and have already invaded and incorporated maternal blood vessels to provide lakes of maternal blood (lacunae). The buds of these trophoblastic cells grow into long, branching fronds called villi, which project into the lakes of blood. As the maternal blood circulates, the villi absorb from it a continuous supply of oxygen and food for the further growth of the embryo.

The amniotic cavity now grows much faster than the yolk sac and as the embryonic disc grows outwards and rolls in on itself lengthways and sideways, the amniotic cavity follows the curving ectodermal layer and eventually encompasses the embryo in a protective sac ending at the body stalk (umbilical cord).

The trophoblast immediately deep to the original attachment of the blastocyst grows very rapidly and develops into the placenta, whereas the trophoblast surrounding the growing embryonic sac and projecting into the cavity of the uterus (the chorion) ceases to grow and function as it moves further away from the source of food and oxygen in the maternal blood. At about the fourth month of pregnancy it comes to lie in contact with the opposite uterine wall with the amnion close behind it. This has the effect of filling the uterus completely at about the fourth month of pregnancy.

ENDODERM (INNER LAYER *of* CELLS)

The growth of the head and tail folds and the rolling over of the ectodermal layer of the embryonic disc produce a tube of endoderm within the developing embryo, largely cut off from but still continuous with the yolk sac. This tube of endoderm forms the primitive alimentary canal. From its upper part will bud off and grow the trachea and the lungs. Further down, the liver and pancreas will also develop from it, and at the tail end of the tube, the bladder, the urethra and in females the lower part of the vagina will appear.

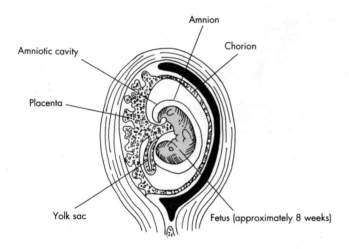

Amnion

Chorion

Amniotic cavity

Placenta

Yolk sac

Fetus (approximately 8 weeks)

Development of the placenta and membranes

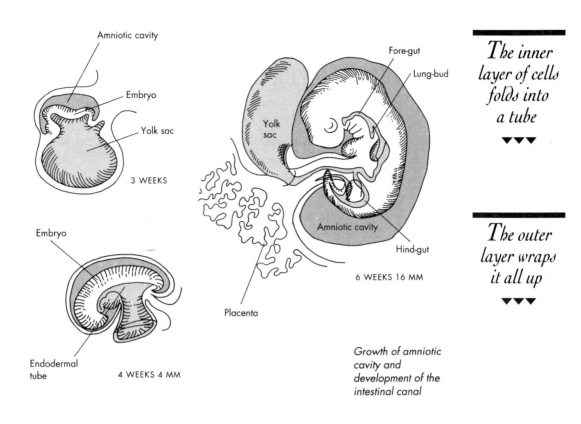

Amniotic cavity

Embryo

Yolk sac

3 WEEKS

Embryo

Endodermal tube

4 WEEKS 4 MM

Fore-gut

Lung-bud

Yolk sac

Amniotic cavity

Hind-gut

6 WEEKS 16 MM

Placenta

Growth of amniotic cavity and development of the intestinal canal

The inner layer of cells folds into a tube

▼▼▼

The outer layer wraps it all up

▼▼▼

ECTODERM (OUTER LAYER *of* CELLS)

The surface layer of cells (ectoderm) of the embryo will produce the whole of the skin including the hair, the nails, the cornea of the eye and the eardrum. In addition, a groove in the ectoderm down the middle of the back of the embryo (the neural groove) will deepen and finally close over to produce the brain and the spinal cord. The middle section of the groove closes over about three weeks after conception and the head and tail segments within the next week. As the brain is developing at this stage, the head end of the embryo grows rapidly.

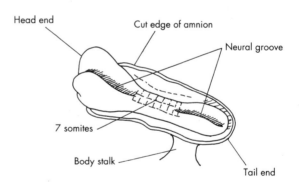

Head end

Cut edge of amnion

Neural groove

7 somites

Body stalk

Tail end

Ectodermal surface of germinal disc 22 days since conception

MESODERM (MIDDLE LAYER *of* CELLS)

About two weeks after fertilisation, another group of cells, the mesoderm, can be seen at the tail end of the embryonic disc. These grow forwards between the ectoderm and the endoderm and backwards into the developing body stalk and the placental villi. Here they form the primitive blood vessels of the embryo and of the villi, for the embryo is now moving further away from its source of food and oxygen and must develop its own circulation and blood cells to carry food and oxygen from the placenta to itself.

Within the embryo, the mesoderm forms a simple system of blood vessels which becomes well established within the next two weeks. About the same time a specialised part of the mesoderm, consisting of heart muscle cells, begins to beat, circulating the embryonic blood back and forth from the embryo to the placenta by way of the body stalk.

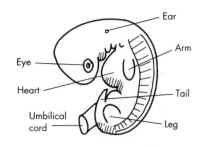

5 weeks since conception
7 weeks amenorrhoea
Crown rump length 9 mm

The mesoderm also lays down specialised cells which will form the muscles, skeleton, ureters, kidneys and most of the internal male and female genital organs.

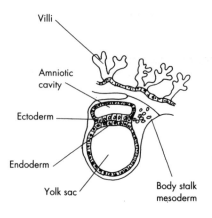

15 days since conception

SEGMENTAL DEVELOPMENT

Along the trunk of the embryo, pairs of segmented areas called somites develop between the 21st and 31st days.

These develop from the mesoderm and will ultimately become the bones of the spinal column, enclosing the spinal cord as the neural groove closes over. Beginning at the head end with four occipital somites, new ones develop progressively downwards until 42 to 44 pairs are formed in the 10 mm long embryo. There are always four occipital and eight cervical and usually 12 thoracic, five lumbar, five sacral and eight to 10 coccygeal pairs of somites. The first occipital and the last seven or eight coccygeal somites stop growing at an early age and disappear. The occipital somites form part of the base of the skull and the remaining ones form the adult vertebrae of the spinal column and their associated muscles.

Most of the bony skeleton is laid down as cartilage, of mesodermal origin, which later develops into mature bone. The bones forming the vault of the skull are membranous rather than cartilagenous in origin, allowing the head to expand rapidly as the brain grows.

So, only six weeks after fertilisation, the embryonic development is such that in a 10 mm long embryo, all of the ultimate organs of the body can be recognised in a primitive form. Within a further two weeks, the embryo has grown to 17 mm, and has assumed a definite human appearance with eyes and ears clearly visible, and the limbs well formed. Embryonic development will be over in a further two weeks and all subsequent changes will be growth in size.

It is during these first eight to 12 weeks of life that the embryo is vulnerable to a variety of outside environmental influences. It is also during this time that any genetic errors will disturb the normal development of the organs, producing certain congenital abnormalities.

FETUS

From the third month onwards, it is customary to change from the word embryo and refer instead to the fetus. A further change, relating to the age of the embryo and fetus, must also be explained at this time. Embryology, which is largely a microscopic study of the early embryo, dates all embryos from the moment of conception. Obstetricians, on the other hand, date fetal age from the only known date, the first day of the last menstrual period. If a woman has normal 28 day cycles, ovulation and conception can be expected to occur 14 days after her last menstrual period. So, when an obstetrician refers to a 14 weeks fetus, he is really saying that it is 14 weeks since the mother's last

The body of the embryo develops segments

▼▼▼

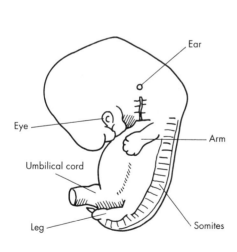

6 weeks since conception
8 weeks amenorrhoea
Crown rump length 12.2 mm

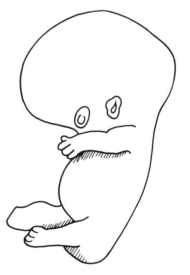

7 weeks since conception
9 weeks amenorrhoea
Crown rump length 17 mm

menstrual period began (referred to as 14 weeks amenorrhoea); in fact, the fetus is only 12 weeks old. All pregnancies are dated in this way.

CONGENITAL ABNORMALITIES

In Australia the incidence of major abnormalities — those which limit normal function—detected at birth is approximately 1 in 75. However, less obvious problems such as heart and kidney abnormalities and some brain disturbances may not appear until later in life. If all these problems, as well as minor defects such as birthmarks and webbed toes are taken into account, the incidence of congenital abnormalities can be as high as 1 in 20. Some problems are more common in certain racial groups. Even within the same racial group there may be variations associated with certain communities or geographical regions.

There are many reasons why these abnormalities may occur. The most likely explanation is that the embryo must first have a genetic predisposition to the abnormality. This is inherited from the parents. Secondly, there has to be exposure to some agent such as a virus or a chemical substance which is capable of producing abnormal development. Finally, contact with such an agent has to occur at the time when the affected organs or limbs are actually developing.

As an example, in the 1960s the sedative drug thalidomide produced limb deformities in some of the offspring of mothers who took the drug at the particular stage of pregnancy when the limbs were developing. However, the majority of women who took the tablets at this critical time did not produce babies with limb deformities: there apparently was no genetic predisposition to defects in these babies. Similarly, only a minority of women who contract German measles (rubella) in the first three months of pregnancy produce infants with the deformities which we know the disease can cause.

Very few drugs are known to cause congenital abnormalities. As a rule, however, it is wisest to avoid drugs during pregnancy unless there is a good reason for taking them. Alcohol, tobacco and marijuana should also be avoided. The period during which drugs or other agents can cause malformations is very short. It is usually over by the eighth week after conception, which is the time when a lot of women are first certain that they are pregnant. However, even at this stage, some anatomical structures may not yet be fully developed, such as the palate, external genitals and brain.

The mother's age also has a bearing on the incidence of abnormalities. They are more likely to occur in babies of girls in their early to mid-teens. Women in their late 30s and early 40s have a higher incidence of chromosomal abnormalities.

Abnormalities related to the age of the mother are almost all due to chromosomal disorders of which Down's Syndrome (mongolism) is by far the most common. Down's syndrome is thought to occur when an egg with an extra chromosome is fertilised. No similar increase in chromosomal abnormalities has yet been observed with increasing paternal age. However, it is known that chromosomes in both men and women are more likely to break as age increases. This breakage can lead to an exchange of fragments between various chromosomes, a process known as translocation. In some instances, translocation of chromosomes may be associated with congenital abnormalities, yet in other instances it occurs in people regarded as perfectly normal.

DIAGNOSING ABNORMALITIES

Some abnormalities can be diagnosed in the first half of pregnancy. However, those due to drugs or viral illnesses are not in this group. The conditions for which a specific diagnostic test is available, are listed below:

a. Women who will be 37 or over at the time of delivery.
b. A woman of any age who, in a previous pregnancy, delivered a child with a chromosomal abnormality.
c. Couples where one partner carries a chromosomal rearrangement (balanced translocation). These couples are usually indentifed because of recurrent miscarriages or the delivery of a child with multiple abnormalities.
d. Couples at risk of producing sons with a genetic abnormality (X-linked). This category includes some forms of muscular dystrophy, a variety of mental retardation, and haemophilia. Each of these

conditions is rare — there is quite often a family history which may be present in several generations.
e. Couples where each partner is a carrier for the same specific genetic defect. The most common condition in this group is cystic fibrosis. In every pregnancy, there is a one in four chance that the fetus will inherit the disease.

There are currently two tests which are available to test fetuses at risk.

Chorionic Villus Sampling (CVS) is the newer of the two tests. It involves taking a small sample from the placenta at between 10 and 12 weeks after the last menstrual period. The procedure can be done either through the cervix with a speculum in the vagina as if a Pap smear was to be taken. CVS can also be done by putting a needle through the abdominal wall. The results take approximately two weeks but for some rare conditions, the answers may not be available for four weeks. The risk of miscarriage following a CVS is around two in 100 patients. This includes all those patients who were going to miscarry anyway. The procedure itself only accounts for a small part of this risk.

Amniocentesis, on the other hand, is usually performed from about 14 weeks after the last menstrual period. This involves taking about a tablespoon of amniotic fluid from around the fetus. A fine needle is inserted through the maternal abdomen and into the amniotic space. As there are less cells in this specimen, the results take slightly longer. The usual time is about three weeks. The same

The risk may increase with increasing maternal age
▼▼▼

The amniotic fluid can yield secrets
▼▼▼

Some disorders are sex-linked
▼▼▼

information will be obtained as for CVS. One extra test is done at amniocentesis for patients whose children are at risk for spina bifida. The miscarriage rate following amniocentesis is around one in 100. Again this includes those patients who were going to miscarry anyway. The procedurally related miscarriage rate is not significantly different between the two tests.

Both procedures are done under ultrasound control and require the woman to have a comfortably full bladder. In both cases she is usually at the hospital for less than one hour and may essentially go about normal activities following the procedure.

If an abnormality is found, then an appointment to a genetics fetal abnormality clinic will be quickly arranged if needed.

Ultrasound examination which is best done at around 18 weeks since the last menstrual period if looking specifically for abnormalities is good at detecting major structural problems. These disorders include some forms of dwarfism, some kidney disorders, some heart defects, and malformations of the skull and spinal column.

When an abnormality is diagnosed later in pregnancy (after 20 weeks), or the fetus is at risk from severe anaemia, then a sample of fetal blood may be required to investigate the problem. This is done under ultrasound control and involves inserting a fine needle into the umbilical cord. It can be done as an outpatient procedure and carries a risk for premature labour or fetal demise of about one in 50 procedures. The risk is related to how unwell the baby is.

Miscarriage
is a common
problem
▼▼▼

If any of these tests reveal an abnormality, the effects which the abnormality would have on the baby and on the parents is explained precisely to both parents. This information is usually given by the doctor who has done the procedures in association with a geneticist or paediatrician. If the parents decide that they wish to have the pregnancy terminated, this is also fully discussed. Following a CVS, termination of pregnancy involves a curettage of the uterus. Termination later in pregnancy may involve a labour. Labour is induced using vaginal tablets containing an artificial prostaglandin. Delivery usually occurs within 24 hours. During this time the mother is in hospital. Termination of pregnancy by either of these means carries only a very small complication rate.

MISCARRIAGE

Miscarriage (spontaneous abortion) is the passage of the fetus and all or part of the placenta during the first 20 weeks after the last menstrual period. After 20 weeks the term 'pre-term birth' applies.

Miscarriage is a very common complication of early pregnancy. Possibly 50 per cent of all conceptions miscarry, most of them in the early stages. The majority go unrecognised, being regarded as late but heavy periods. The risk of miscarriage is highest immediately after conception and implantation, and diminishes as the pregnancy progresses. By far the most common cause of early miscarriage is fetal abnormality and it has been estimated that 70 per cent of miscarriages occurring before 12 weeks are associated with chromosomal problems.

The first sign of miscarriage is vaginal bleeding, which may not necessarily be heavy. Frequently it is painless and is unrelated to activity. At this stage it is called a 'threatened' miscarriage and usually the bleeding subsides and the pregnancy continues normally. There is no specific treatment for this condition and it is doubtful if bed rest is of any benefit. Fortunately, among babies born to mothers who 'threatened' to miscarry there is no higher incidence of malformation than among babies whose mothers had no bleeding early in pregnancy.

In some instances vaginal bleeding continues, accompanied by abdominal cramps as the cervix opens up. At this stage the miscarriage is regarded as 'inevitable'. Sometimes the embryo and placenta are passed completely and the bleeding stops. More commonly, the placenta remains and the bleeding continues. In this situation, known as 'incomplete' miscarriage, admission to hospital and emptying of the uterus by curettage under general anaesthetic are required to stop the bleeding and prevent infection.

Occasionally, after what appears to be quite minimal bleeding the fetus dies but the woman does not miscarry. This condition is described as a 'missed' abortion. The diagnosis may be difficult to make as the uterus remains enlarged, although other symptoms of pregnancy usually disappear rapidly. If the diagnosis of missed abortion is suspected, it can be confirmed easily by an ultrasonic examination. Most doctors would then recommend curettage of the uterus.

Mothers with Rhesus negative blood should receive an injection of anti-D gamma-globulin following the miscarriage in order to lessen the risk of developing immunity to Rhesus positive blood cells absorbed from the embryo. If such immunisation occurs it can affect future pregnancies (see Chapter 7: *Is there something wrong, doctor?*).

There is a small group of women who have little difficulty in conceiving, but who have difficulty carrying a pregnancy to viability. One in 10 such couples will have one member with a chromosomal rearrangement (translocation) and one in every 10 women who miscarry repeatedly will have a congenital abnormality of the uterus. Women with auto-immune diseases are known to have a risk of miscarriage as high as 50 per cent and the consumption of one drink of alcohol every day is sufficient to double the basic rate of miscarriage. In the days when doctors understood very little about the hormonal circumstances of pregnancy, it was believed that a 'hormone deficiency' could be responsible for recurrent pregnancy losses. Nowadays this is known not to be true and no normal pregnancy has ever been shown to have been lost because of any hormone deficiency. In addition to hormonal therapy having repetitively been shown to be of no benefit, the taking of these powerful sex steroids is not without risk to the fetus, and should be avoided.

A miscarriage may 'threaten'

▼▼▼

or become 'inevitable' or be 'incomplete'

▼▼▼

or be 'missed'

▼▼▼

Occasionally an immunological cause is suspected in couples in whom all investigations reveal no abnormality. Recent studies have shown that immunotherapy, whereby women receive injections of their partners white blood cells, results in a higher success rate in subsequent pregnancies than when such immunisation is not performed.

In approximately 50 per cent of recurrent miscarriages, no obvious cause can be found and the success in subsequent pregnancies may be signficantly enhanced by an optimistic approach from the medical attendants involved.

OTHER CAUSES *of* BLEEDING *in* EARLY PREGNANCY

Sometimes bleeding in early pregnancy is not associated with miscarriage. Bleeding from the cervix can occur following intercourse or even from straining when constipated, as the cervix is much softer during pregnancy and bleeds easily.

Vaginal bleeding may also be associated with an ectopic pregnancy. This is a situation where the fertilised egg implants somewhere other than in the cavity of the uterus. Most ectopic pregnancies occur in the Fallopian tubes. The bleeding is often preceded by pain low in the abdomen which may be quite severe. This situation occurs in one in every 200 pregnancies. If left untreated, heavy bleeding frequently occurs when the tube ruptures, resulting in intense pain and sometimes severe shock. For this reason it is important to seek advice if an episode of lower abdominal pain is followed by vaginal bleeding. If an ectopic pregnancy is diagnosed or if it is suspected, admission to hospital is required. If the diagnosis is obvious an operation will be performed to remove the portion of the tube which contains the embryo. When the diagnosis is in doubt, an operation called a laparoscopy is performed: a very thin telescope-like instrument is inserted into the mother's abdomen so that the uterus and tubes can be inspected. If the diagnosis is then confirmed, an operation is performed to remove the embryo from the tube.

A very rare cause of bleeding in pregnancy is hydatidiform mole. This is a disorder due to abnormal development of the placenta and it occurs in approximately one in 800 pregnancies in Australia. The placental tissue forms little sacs (vesicles) which rapidly enlarge. Neither amniotic fluid nor the membranes which usually surround the fluid are formed. In almost all instances there is no embryo; it dies early on because of an inadequate blood supply. The amount of bleeding can vary considerably and the patient may even pass some of the vesicles through the vagina. The uterus is often larger than one would expect. The diagnosis can be confirmed by examining the urine: unusually high concentrations of hCG (human chorionic gonadotrophin), the placental hormone used to diagnose pregnancy, are commonly found. When the level of this hormone is very high, the woman often experiences the symptoms of early pregnancy to a far greater degree than otherwise. Nausea and vomiting may be quite pronounced. The diagnosis can be confirmed by ultrasound where a typical picture of numerous vesicles may be seen. If a diagnosis of hydatidiform mole is made, the mother is admitted to hospital. Under a general anaesthetic the cervix is dilated and the mole is removed from the uterus by suction and curettage. Pregnancy should not be contemplated for at least six months after treatment for a hydatidiform mole, and during this time regular checks of the hCG level in the blood will be carried out. The reason for this is that sometimes women who have hydatidiform moles may subsequently develop a tumour called choriocarcinoma which fortunately responds readily to modern drug treatment. If a woman has a hydatidiform mole or even a choriocarcinoma it does not mean that she cannot have children in the future.

MULTIPLE PREGNANCY

Twin pregnancy is said to occur in one in every 80 pregnancies amongst people of European descent. The incidence differs between racial groups, being less common among Asian people and more common in Negro populations.

The incidence of triplets is one in 6400 (80^2), quadruplets one in 512 000 (80^3), and so on. These figures do not include multiple births due to drugs taken to induce ovulation. The incidence of multiple pregnancy is greater amongst women who have taken such drugs than one would otherwise expect.

Twin pregnancies may arise either from one egg (uniovular) or two eggs (binovular). Triplets and above usually result from simultaneous fertilisation of three or more eggs.

With uniovular twins, one ovum only is fertilised but early in development it splits to form two embryos. However, in many cases the placenta is shared. Such twins are also described as 'monozygous' or 'identical'.

Binovular twins occur when two eggs are fertilised and two embryos and two placentas develop. These twins, often called fraternal twins, are not identical and may be of different sex. Binovular twins are commonly found in different generations of the mother's family and appear to be more common in women over 35 years of age. There are no such obvious relationships for uniovular twins.

More than one baby
▼▼▼

Identical twins
▼▼▼

Fraternal twins
▼▼▼

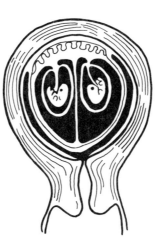

Identical twins

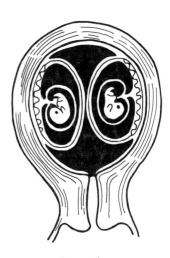

Fraternal twins

CHAPTER 3

WHY DO I FEEL LIKE THIS...

Emotional Aspects of Pregnancy

Pregnancy does not just happen to a body, it happens to a person. That person usually finds it is a time of changed feelings, which although exciting can also cause anxiety.

While many an expectant mother may say it isn't easy being pregnant, there are others who find it a happy and satisfying time when they feel at peace with the world and fulfilled in their womanhood.

Each woman faces every situation with her unique personality, expectations, values, relationships and domestic situation. She will respond to pregnancy in her own way. In her first pregnancy especially, she may need to compare her feelings

Pregnancy can have some unexpected effects
▼▼▼

Everyone is different
▼▼▼

with other people's, to see if her experiences are 'normal'. Suddenly, however, everyone seems to be an expert on the subject and it is very difficult to know what is 'normal' especially when well-meaning friends, relatives or women at work will insist that whatever happened to them was the 'right thing'.

There is no need to stop listening, but it is important for every woman to remind herself that she is a unique human being, and that her feelings are important whether they are the same as Aunt Joan's or not. It is normal to feel elated and it is normal to feel depressed. It is normal to feel highly sensitive and tearful and it is normal to feel calm and serene. It is also normal to experience all these feelings at different times.

HISTORY

Modern woman faces a situation quite unlike the experiences of her great-grandmother, grandmother and mother. The rituals and mythology that have been slowly disappearing from childbirth in the western world since the turn of the century are now all but gone. They have been replaced with scientific and medical facts, which can often seem cold and impersonal and leave the pregnant woman feeling not only vulnerable but even distressed and guilty about the myriad of feelings and emotions she may have. Women are now often expected to believe that pregnancy and childbirth are natural events, with no room for drama, and that every woman should be able to handle them with composure as she looks forward to experiencing a warm and deeply personal relationship with her baby. In fact, this is not always possible.

In years gone by, childbirth was a matter for women alone. It was handled by mothers, sisters, aunts, cousins, and midwives with the doctor occasionally getting a look in. A woman usually lived close to her family and once she married, pregnancy was a matter of course. Her pregnancy involved certain rituals, which, if she performed them correctly, she believed would ensure a healthy child. Thus arose the old wives' tales.

She accepted with contentment or resignation her role in life as someone's daughter, wife, mother and grandmother. She knew she was probably destined for many pregnancies and equally that not all her children would survive to adulthood.

How things have changed. Feminist activity has ensured that the woman is recognised as a person in her own right. Women are now educated, hold senior executive or political positions, own property, can initiate divorce, and of great importance, control their reproduction.

IT HAPPENS *to* TWO PEOPLE

The Australian woman today faces pregnancy and motherhood as never before. With her mother, sisters and even grandmother likely to be holding jobs themselves or living some distance away, she relies more heavily than ever on her partner, her doctor, and the advice of 'expert' friends.

More than ever before, a baby is born to a couple rather than to a woman. Father has been involved in the pregnancy in a way men before him have not. The pregnancy was probably planned and decided on together. He takes part in visits for check-ups, preparation for labour and parenthood classes, and eventually in the delivery of the child. He becomes responsible, perhaps for the first time since marriage, for financially supporting his partner and providing for their material needs from his salary alone.

For many couples, having a child is an expression of their shared love and of their desire to grow through nurturing another human. Their relationship is expanded and deepened by sharing the joys and the woes of pregnancy and approaching parenthood. All this requires an important ingredient in the relationship: open and honest communication. The ability to talk about what each is feeling, knowing the other partner will accept and respect the feelings, even if she or he cannot understand them, and the capacity to compromise, are essential ingredients.

EMOTIONAL REACTIONS

How a woman first reacts to being pregnant depends on whether this is, or is not, what she wants. If the pregnancy is unwanted, the first few weeks can be a time of intense distress and anxiety until she makes a decision about the future. Once this is resolved, she is free to continue the pregnancy with a greater possibility of enjoying the experience.

If a pregnancy is much longed for and wanted, a woman's first reaction is intense happiness, mingled perhaps with a feeling of anti-climax. She may be rather annoyed that her body does not yet look pregnant and be quite impatient for it to do so. If the physical aspects of early pregnancy are particularly uncomfortable or cause illness, a woman may become anxious for all to go well.

When the tiredness and nausea of early pregnancy pass and more obvious swelling of the tummy begins, there often comes a feeling of contentment and well-being. The first movements of the baby can be a time of exultation and, for some women, a confirmation of the pregnancy. With this there often comes a feeling of urgency to get things done and organised, a need to start gathering things for the baby and preparing the place for the baby. It is from this point that a woman is likely to start talking to the baby. For other women, however, a baby will not be real until it is born and can be seen. To these women all the preparations can be somewhat dreamlike.

Interestingly, a few women experience a marked change in character during pregnancy. The usually anxious, sensitive woman may become quite serene, calmly accepting whatever goes on around her. A usually unflappable woman can find herself suddenly becoming irritable, upset and tearful. Thus some women are at their best when pregnant and others really dislike it. These changes can be disconcerting not only for the woman herself but also for her partner.

The last few weeks of pregnancy are usually a time of real physical discomfort and there is a strong desire for the whole thing to be over. There have been months of waiting and preparing and all that is missing is the baby. The woman is ready and anxious to move from being pregnant to being a mother.

The emotional effects of pregnancy vary from month to month

▼ ▼ ▼

CHANGES

The physical aspects of pregnancy can be demoralising. Feeling very ill for the first few months, having a bladder that never seems empty, being unable to sleep, having an object pounding away inside, getting hotter and more tired than usual, developing pimples, feeling fat and lumpy, or looking in the mirror and thinking 'yuk' can leave a woman feeling plain fed up.

Other people's attitudes to pregnant women can be disconcerting. It can be irritating when others expect that the pregnant woman only wants to talk about childbirth and babies. It can seem as if the pregnant woman has lost her individuality and her mind, becoming part of the amorphous group of mothers-to-be that can be patronised, advised and smiled at indulgently. While such reactions are changing in the health care area this is not necessarily the case in the general community. Indeed some people feel quite ill at ease with a pregnant woman.

There are a growing number of women who defer motherhood until their late 30s. By this time a woman is characteristically in control of her life and has an established job or career. Such women can have an expectation that they will handle the pregnancy in a mature fashion. Any unexpected complications or feelings in pregnancy, and the demands of motherhood can lead to feelings of inadequacy. For those who plan to leave the workforce temporarily, there is an added need to resolve strong conflicting emotional needs.

This is not an easy task for women who usually make logical analyses and decisions. All these changes make a woman feel different physically and emotionally both from other people and from her former self. Somehow the normal pattern of life and relating to others is out of balance. She must adjust to this but it is not always easy because she is not entirely sure how she is supposed to react, especially if she does not feel like the ideal pictures of expectant mothers in magazines.

MOOD SWINGS

Today, she feels wonderful, relaxed, happy with the world and savouring the very personal joy of having a life growing within her. By the same evening she may be feeling tearful and depressed for apparently no reason. Whatever her partner says does nothing to make her feel better and she finds she bursts into tears for no reason and becomes irritable over small things. Pregnant women are quite likely to 'make mountains out of molehills'.

Mood swings are very common in pregnancy. The body is undergoing great changes and these swings, which can occur from day to day or hour to hour, are in early pregnancy probably related to hormone changes. They are generally mild and can be handled with ease. However, they can be severe, or be exacerbated by external pressures. A woman who is involved in moving house or worrying about financial problems, for example, is liable to become more

It would be a lot easier to sit on an egg
▼▼▼

Pregnant women can be upset very easily
▼▼▼

depressed, irritable and tearful than one who is not experiencing these extra pressures. These changes in a woman can be alarming for her partner, who may find he is living with quite a different person from the woman with whom he started out. Coming home after a busy day to a tearful, irritable partner, who does not know what is upsetting her, can be a lot to take. Again, communication and mutual respect for feelings become essential in maintaining a happy relationship. Many a marriage has been broken by a pregnancy and by the inability of a couple to share their feelings about it.

SENSITIVITY and APPETITE

Many a pregnant woman is surprised by her heightened sensitivity to what is happening around her. She can get great joy from things she had perhaps not noticed before, perhaps a sunny morning or a bird's song.

This sensitivity can also affect her normal likes and dislikes so that she cannot bear the smell of coffee or cigarette smoke or the taste of alcohol, and may even develop some bizarre cravings. It may also affect her sexual appetite, making her either more or less desirous of sexual relations with her partner, and she may have more or less intense physical reactions during intercourse. Some women experience orgasm only during pregnancy, others lose their sexual desire and do not wish to have intercourse at all. Like all the other changes of pregnancy, this can be

confusing both to the woman and to her partner. Having these changed feelings does not mean there is anything wrong with her, but unless she tells her partner what is happening, misunderstandings can arise and cause problems. Partners will need to find different ways of meeting each other's needs and pregnancy can open the door to sexual experimentation and bring a new dimension to their relationship.

DREAMS and FANTASIES

It is common for a pregnant woman, especially in the later stages of pregnancy, to have vivid dreams that might be quite horrific. They are often related to babies or children and may involve mutilation, disastrous accidents and other frightening events. Sometimes such dreams recur night after night.

These dreams are probably due to the very reasonable anxiety most women feel about the outcome of their pregnancy. Although this anxiety about the prospective baby is present throughout the entire pregnancy, it may heighten in the last weeks. It is a common and understandable feeling and even if it does result in bad dreams cannot have any effect on the unborn child. Dreams about deformed children or accidents to children or loved ones do not make such things happen and are not an omen that they will happen. In the same way, experiencing an emotional trauma such as the death of a relative or close friend will not affect the baby.

'I've stopped smoking, why can't you?'
▼▼▼

Dreams don't come true, but fantasies are fun
▼▼▼

In her waking hours a woman may find herself fantasising about the future, seeing herself in her role as a new mother. Unlike some dreams, these are usually pleasant episodes. The baby she pictures is likely to look like a small version of her or her partner, very attractive and of the happy disposition and plump good health of those little angels in advertisements. These fantasies are the way in which a woman mentally practises being a mother and prepares herself emotionally for that role. Inevitably when a new experience is anticipated, a great amount of energy and thought is given to considering how one will behave in the new situation. Impending motherhood and fatherhood are no different.

Sometimes thinking about being a mother can cause anxiety. This is usually because of some unhappy or unsatisfactory past mothering experience. On the whole, humans learn how to behave by imitation. Children therefore grow up to be like their parents and often raise their own children the way they themselves were raised. If a woman had a happy, secure and loving childhood, she has a good model to build on. If she did not have such a background, she may feel anxious about being a mother; she may well know what she wants for her baby but be unsure of how to achieve it.

She may have had an essentially happy childhood but have had other negative mothering experiences. The eldest daughter of a very large family, for example, may have been required in her early years to stay at home and care for younger children when she would have preferred to be out playing with her friends. So mothering for her may be associated with those old repressed feelings of resentment and anger. Identifying the cause of any such anxiety can help to overcome it.

Occasionally women are concerned about their child being born on a certain day such as the anniversary of the death of a much loved relative. They may be concerned about the child being born under a certain astrological sign. Some cultures believe that certain years are good luck.

There is no proof that any of these factors have the desired effects. However, if parents persist in treating the child in a particular way because of a coincidence of birth, then their fears may be realised — because of their attitudes. All children are individuals in their own right and must be thought of as such.

Dreams and fantasies during pregnancy play a part in preparing a woman for her new role. They are not, however, reality, and, whatever fears she may have, a woman is most likely to have a normal, healthy baby.

ADJUSTMENT

Each pregnancy requires the partners to do some adjusting in their lives, especially with their first child. Resisting the need to change can bring problems. One thing is certain: life will never be the same again.

For most couples there is a financial change to be made. This can cause concern, particularly in a society in which families are

Mothering behaviour needs a model
▼▼▼

Some babies have to be born on 29 February
▼▼▼

Making changes may not be easy
▼▼▼

predominantly two-income, especially during a first pregnancy. Many prospective fathers think they should not worry their pregnant partners about financial matters and they suffer the worries alone. Many a pregnant woman finds it hard to accept financial dependence and resents asking for money. Like all aspects of pregnancy, plans for financial arrangements must be shared.

Unexpected pregnancies, often as a result of failed contraception, also require adjustment. Often other children are at school, the mother may be working and she may see herself at a different stage in her life.

Such families may have no real financial, housing or other worries and to make it harder to talk through her negative feelings, everyone else is delighted! A big emotional shift is necessary to come to accept this pregnancy and for some professional counselling is necessary.

Many couples consider moving house prior to a baby's birth. Remember, though, that this is a traumatic event. There is the search, the anxiety, and the effort of actually moving. Although the end result is perhaps a place more suitable for a baby, it also often represents a new neighbourhood and new friends and more adjustments to make.

After the baby arrives, a woman will devote most of her time and energy to the child. Having helpful neighbours, knowing the local facilities and feeling secure are important factors in counteracting the feelings of loneliness, lack of stimulation and anxiety of which increasing numbers of mothers

Don't plan to move house

▼▼▼

complain. For the woman moving into a new neighbourhood or giving up a job that has prevented her getting to know her community, those weeks before the baby is born can be very profitably spent in making new friends and finding out just what happens and is available in the area. The local newspapers and Baby Health Centre are good beginnings for this new adventure.

MEN

To a man, pregnancy and childbirth may seem to be so much women's work, and in the past this view was reinforced by the way they were handled. Today, however, prospective fathers are increasingly taking a more active part in these important episodes in their partner's life, as now there is greater understanding of the value to the child of a close relationship with both his parents from the earliest possible time.

As a result, a man is now expected to understand and accept his partner's changing shape and moods, to assist and support her on an equal basis in her daily tasks and, in short, to do almost everything except give birth. His own father is likely to be quite mystified by this behaviour, as he is most unlikely to have been subject to the same expectations. Therefore, what model does a man have to follow? He is undoubtedly a pioneer in this changing image of the male role.

It is perhaps no wonder a fellow feels somewhat confused at times about how to react and what to do. It is difficult when a normally calm woman starts crying without warning and then cannot say why; when her sexual appetite increases or decreases; when she wants the baby's nursery decorated immediately and he knows there are still months to go; or when that growing tummy turns him off rather than on.

It can be annoying when no one can talk of anything other than babies; it can be worrying contemplating how to afford the next instalment on the car. Yet father is supposed to be 'strong' and shoulder these things. It is perfectly understandable if a man withdraws and becomes edgy and irritable or seems to need an extra drink with 'the boys' after work.

Most men feel elated at the prospect of being a father and are as keen as their partners to enjoy the planning and anticipation. They may feel hesitant about what to do but are usually pleased to be asked to share and they gain satisfaction from making a positive and helpful contribution. A woman may get much more happiness and satisfaction from a pregnancy if it is enjoyed with the one other person who has an intimate investment in the outcome.

To sum up, pregnancy is a special time. It may be full of conflicting feelings, some anxieties and much happiness. When expecting their first child, it is probably the last time a couple will be alone for some years.

It is a valuable time that can show a profit. This will occur if a couple take notice of what is happening to them, respect each other's needs, thoughts and feelings, and plan together in a realistic way for the future. There is a bit of magic in pregnancy but a lot of hard work.

Pregnancy is special...

▼▼▼

but it's hard work too

▼▼▼

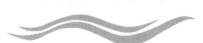

CHAPTER 4

...AND THIS?

Physical Aspects of Pregnancy

Once pregnancy commences, there will be inevitable physical changes in the mother's body, not only in the growing uterus, but in many distant organs as well.

These changes will produce various effects which are a normal part of pregnancy but which the mother may interpret as signs of illness. Knowing these normal changes is necessary for a correct understanding of pregnancy.

Physical changes are normal

▼▼▼

NO PERIODS (AMENORRHOEA)

This is usually the first clue that a pregnancy is under way. Periods may be delayed for lots of reasons, such as fear of pregnancy, stopping taking the Pill, or because of the stress of travelling. However, the usual reason a period does not arrive when expected is because conception took place some two weeks previously.

Periods will be absent during pregnancy and afterwards may not return for many months for a variety of reasons (see Chapter 15: *I didn't know it would be like this*).

PREGNANCY TESTS

With some exceptions, the reason a period does not come is because the tiny developing embryo gives a hormonal signal to the body not to menstruate and therefore expel it from the uterus. It is possible to measure this signalling hormone, hCG (human chorionic gonadotrophin), in both blood and urine.

A urine test can be done by you, your chemist, your doctor or at a hospital. These tests have become more accurate in the last few years. A urine test may be performed one to two days after a missed period and if positive will signify the presence of a pregnancy. A negative test does not mean you are not pregnant as the level of hormone may be too low to detect. The specimen of urine tested should be the first of the day because it is more concentrated and so contains the highest hormone levels.

A blood test can be taken any time of the day and will give an accurate result as early as five days after conception and so may be positive even before a period is missed.

Talking in months can be inaccurate
▼▼▼

ESTIMATED DATE *of* DELIVERY (EDD)

The average length of time from the beginning of the last period until the baby is born is 283 days (just over 40 weeks).

GESTATION TABLE

Find the date of the first day of your last normal menstrual period in the top line of each row. The estimated date of delivery is the date beneath this, assuming your menstrual cycles are regular and last 28 days.

JANUARY	1	2	3	4	5	6	7	8	9	10	11	12	13	14	15	16	17	18	19	20	21	22	23	24	25	26	27	28	29	30	31
OCT/NOV	11	12	13	14	15	16	17	18	19	20	21	22	23	24	25	26	27	28	29	30	31	1	2	3	4	5	6	7	8	9	10
FEBRUARY	1	2	3	4	5	6	7	8	9	10	11	12	13	14	15	16	17	18	19	20	21	22	23	24	25	26	27	28			
NOV/DEC	11	12	13	14	15	16	17	18	19	20	21	22	23	24	25	26	27	28	29	30	1	2	3	4	5	6	7	8			
MARCH	1	2	3	4	5	6	7	8	9	10	11	12	13	14	15	16	17	18	19	20	21	22	23	24	25	26	27	28	29	30	31
DEC/JAN	9	10	11	12	13	14	15	16	17	18	19	20	21	22	23	24	25	26	27	28	29	30	31	1	2	3	4	5	6	7	8
APRIL	1	2	3	4	5	6	7	8	9	10	11	12	13	14	15	16	17	18	19	20	21	22	23	24	25	26	27	28	29	30	
JAN/FEB	9	10	11	12	13	14	15	16	17	18	19	20	21	22	23	24	25	26	27	28	29	30	31	1	2	3	4	5	6	7	
MAY	1	2	3	4	5	6	7	8	9	10	11	12	13	14	15	16	17	18	19	20	21	22	23	24	25	26	27	28	29	30	31
FEB/MAR	8	9	10	11	12	13	14	15	16	17	18	19	20	21	22	23	24	25	26	27	28	1	2	3	4	5	6	7	8	9	10
JUNE	1	2	3	4	5	6	7	8	9	10	11	12	13	14	15	16	17	18	19	20	21	22	23	24	25	26	27	28	29	30	
MAR/APRIL	11	12	13	14	15	16	17	18	19	20	21	22	23	24	25	26	27	28	29	30	31	1	2	3	4	5	6	7	8	9	
JULY	1	2	3	4	5	6	7	8	9	10	11	12	13	14	15	16	17	18	19	20	21	22	23	24	25	26	27	28	29	30	31
APR/MAY	10	11	12	13	14	15	16	17	18	19	20	21	22	23	24	25	26	27	28	29	30	1	2	3	4	5	6	7	8	9	10
AUGUST	1	2	3	4	5	6	7	8	9	10	11	12	13	14	15	16	17	18	19	20	21	22	23	24	25	26	27	28	29	30	31
MAY/JUNE	11	12	13	14	15	16	17	18	19	20	21	22	23	24	25	26	27	28	29	30	31	1	2	3	4	5	6	7	8	9	10
SEPTEMBER	1	2	3	4	5	6	7	8	9	10	11	12	13	14	15	16	17	18	19	20	21	22	23	24	25	26	27	28	29	30	
JUNE/JULY	11	12	13	14	15	16	17	18	19	20	21	22	23	24	25	26	27	28	29	30	1	2	3	4	5	6	7	8	9	10	
OCTOBER	1	2	3	4	5	6	7	8	9	10	11	12	13	14	15	16	17	18	19	20	21	22	23	24	25	26	27	28	29	30	31
JULY/AUG	11	12	13	14	15	16	17	18	19	20	21	22	23	24	25	26	27	28	29	30	31	1	2	3	4	5	6	7	8	9	10
NOVEMBER	1	2	3	4	5	6	7	8	9	10	11	12	13	14	15	16	17	18	19	20	21	22	23	24	25	26	27	28	29	30	
AUG/SEPT	11	12	13	14	15	16	17	18	19	20	21	22	23	24	25	26	27	28	29	30	31	1	2	3	4	5	6	7	8	9	
DECEMBER	1	2	3	4	5	6	7	8	9	10	11	12	13	14	15	16	17	18	19	20	21	22	23	24	25	26	27	28	29	30	31
SEPT/OCT	10	11	12	13	14	15	16	17	18	19	20	21	22	23	24	25	26	27	28	29	30	1	2	3	4	5	6	7	8	9	10

Midwives and doctors talk in weeks rather than months in relation to pregnancy because it is more accurate. The problem in counting in months is that lunar months, that is, 28 days or four weeks, are not the same length as calendar months.

Many doctors count up the days for complete accuracy. A simple way to estimate the dates of delivery is to count 10 days from the beginning of the last period and then add nine calendar months. For example, if the period started on 9 February, the expected date of delivery is 19 November (10 days + 9 months). These calculations are only reliable for women with a regular 28 day cycle. If a woman's cycle is longer she must add the number of days her cycle is in excess of 28 days to her EDD. If the cycle is shorter than 28 days she subtracts the difference.

Just as not everyone is 163 cm tall (average female height), so it follows that not all babies arrive on the estimated date. Only five per cent of women have their babies actually on the predicted date, but 80 per cent give birth 10 days either side of their EDD.

MORNING SICKNESS (NAUSEA)

Morning sickness often occurs in the first weeks of pregnancy, but usually finishes by 12 weeks.

Nausea first thing in the morning may often be prevented by eating a dry biscuit or toast half an hour before getting out of bed. Sickness during the day is often relieved by eating. Try a piece of fruit, some barley sugar or flat lemonade or dry ginger ale. If the feeling persists, try eating small simple meals especially cold foods such as sandwiches, salads or plain biscuits with cheese, every few hours instead of your bigger meals. Avoid spicy and fatty foods, and foods with strong tastes and smells. Try not to miss meals altogether, and attempt to eat something as not eating at all will usually make your nausea worse. If nausea persists you should seek help from your doctor. Return to a good eating pattern as soon as you can.

A partner needs to be especially sensitive to a woman's needs at this time by preparing meals or providing an early morning cup of black tea to help overcome the nausea.

Apart from dietary adjustment, vitamin B6 (pyridoxine) 100 mgs night and morning is of help with nausea and for more troublesome cases there are safe and effective drugs available.

Occasional vomiting may be disturbing to the mother, but it does not harm the baby. However, excessive vomiting when nothing can be kept down is the time to consult the doctor or clinic. Sometimes admission to hospital for intravenous fluid therapy is necessary. This treatment cures the condition by resting the stomach and restoring the fluid balance.

BREAST CHANGES

Breasts are particularly sensitive to the hormonal changes of pregnancy, especially during the first pregnancy.

Some women will already have noticed similar changes in their breasts in the days immediately before their periods.

During early pregnancy the breasts often tingle around the nipple and veins appear on the surface. Later on, the pink skin around the nipple area (areola) darkens and small lumps, called Montgomery's tubercles, appear around its edge. Increasing size and tenseness make the breasts feel heavy. If they are bumped accidentally they may feel very tender.

Milk production does not usually occur until after the baby is born, although a milky fluid (colostrum) often appears unexpectedly from the breasts during the last three months of pregnancy.

A maternity bra is a good idea from as early as 12 weeks not only for comfort but also to help retain breast shape after the baby has been weaned. If breast enlargement is excessive in the early part of pregnancy, a maternity bra may be needed even sooner.

FREQUENCY

This is probably one of the most annoying symptoms of pregnancy. Quite early on, many women often experience the feeling of a very full bladder; this is thought to be due to the increased local blood supply around the bladder, caused by pregnancy.

In addition, the kidneys may produce more urine during pregnancy, so there is more to be passed. Frequency often eases during the middle portion of the pregnancy, only to return towards the end when the baby's head 'engages', thus diminishing the amount of urine that the bladder can hold (see Chapter 6: *Everybody tells me something different*).

FATIGUE

The inbuilt reaction of the body to tire easily during pregnancy is nature's way of ensuring that a woman gets the extra rest she needs in order to be able to nourish the baby both day and night, through the placenta before it is born and through the breast milk afterwards. It is a normal reaction and one should therefore react sensibly to it.

Being tired is so common that women who have already had children may know they are pregnant again just because of this washed-out feeling.

Although a feeling of being 'drained' is normal, if excessive it can be a symptom of anaemia. This is the reason why the doctor checks the blood count early in pregnancy, and may prescribe iron tablets (see Chapter 5: *Is everything alright?*).

It is important to avoid too many social engagements. Working overtime may be even more tiring especially as the pregnancy progresses. It is a mistake for anyone to think they are indispensable at work. If it is financially possible, most pregnant women benefit from stopping work about two months before the baby is due, because extra rest is essential at the end of pregnancy.

'I used to be 32A'

▼▼▼

A full bladder is a common feeling

▼▼▼

Feeling tired is normal

▼▼▼

FAINTING and DIZZY SPELLS

These are very common symptoms in early pregnancy and usually disappear at the same time as nausea does.

The reason for them appears to be that at times insufficient blood is returned to the heart and this in turn deprives the brain of blood and therefore oxygen, so that unless you sit or lie down you will faint. This situation is particularly aggravated in hot weather and in stuffy rooms. It is also very common for a woman to feel light-headed or dizzy but then not actually faint. To try and avoid this, do not get too hot, hungry or hassled.

In late pregnancy, faintness or sickness may occur when lying flat on your back. In this case, roll on to your side, wiggle your toes and the faintness will rapidly disappear (see Chapter 6: *Everybody tells me something different*).

MUCUS DISCHARGE

An increase in normal vaginal discharge is an almost universal symptom. Like most other changes of pregnancy, this comes about because of altered hormone levels and also because of the increased blood supply to the pelvis.

Fortunately, it is not usually heavy enough to cause embarrassment. Some women do prefer to wear a pad, although for most this is unnecessary.

This discharge is not irritating. It is usually clear and does not have an unpleasant odour.

If the discharge changes colour and there is associated itchiness around the vaginal entrance, it is most likely that thrush (monilia) has developed. Thrush is more common during pregnancy than at other times. The treatment is just the same, pregnant or not, and as the drugs used are applied locally and not absorbed into the body, they cannot harm your baby.

HUNGER, WEIGHT GAIN and PICA

There are few things pregnant women become more obsessed with than their weight. Their obsession is rivalled only by that of some doctors and midwives. It is normal for a pregnant woman to gain weight throughout pregnancy; and usually a woman puts on 10 to 13 kg during her pregnancy.

Low calorie diets are sometimes prescribed if weight gain is thought to be excessive but they may be harmful to the baby's development. A sensible balanced diet, spread over the day, helps digestion and gives mother and baby all the food they need (see Chapter 5: *Is everything alright?*).

There are much more important things to discuss during prenatal visits than weight.

Pica (eating highly inappropriate things) is quite a common symptom during pregnancy, and probably everybody has a favourite story about it. Things such as wall plaster and cold Chinese food do not matter particularly. However, some substances may be potentially harmful, so unusual cravings should be checked with your doctor.

STRETCH MARKS (STRIAE)

During pregnancy, these marks in the skin occur mostly on the abdomen, and for some women also on the breasts and the upper thighs. Skin is able to stretch and retract within certain limits. When these limits are exceeded, the elastic fibres of the skin rupture and the site of the rupture is a stretch mark which initially is purple in colour. The marks fade to white after the birth, but never disappear entirely. High hormonal levels also contribute to stretch marks.

Women particularly susceptible to stretch marks are those overweight before the pregnancy, those who gain a large amount of weight during pregnancy, and those with a multiple pregnancy and therefore a bigger uterus stretching the skin of the abdomen.

To limit the appearance of stretch marks, avoid excessive weight gain, keep the skin moist and supple, and maintain good posture with abdominal support (muscle control and a girdle) to limit protrusion of the abdomen. However, these measures will not totally prevent the appearance of stretch marks in all women.

ABDOMINAL ENLARGEMENT

As the pregnant uterus enlarges, it extends up out of the pelvis. However, even before this occurs, the abdomen becomes distended and it is no longer possible to wear slacks or jeans. This initial swelling is due to expansion of the bowel by wind; later, however, it is due to the uterus and the baby inside it.

After the first 12 weeks the uterus can be felt just above the pubic hairline as a soft ball. It continues to enlarge until, with about four weeks to go, it has reached right up to the ribs. Fortunately, at this stage the baby's head usually descends into the pelvis and the woman does not feel as heavy. This sensation, not surprisingly, is called lightening.

Some women worry a great deal if they do not 'show'. The only way to see how big a baby is and how far the pregnancy has advanced is to feel (palpate) the baby. The better the tone of her abdominal muscles, and the trimmer a woman looks, the less advanced her pregnancy appears.

There are many speciality clothes shops for pregnant women and a smart outfit does wonders for morale. But of course you will only wear them a few times, so try to borrow or make your own clothes.

'I can't wear jeans'
▼ ▼ ▼

Skin Changes

Again, hormones are the culprit. Some women notice their complexion becomes blotchy during pregnancy, and they may have noticed similar changes before their periods.

Women who already have acne may find that during pregnancy the condition becomes more noticeable or, conversely, that it improves. The reason for these contradictions is not known.

The best treatment for acne during pregnancy is to wash well with mild soap and then apply an astringent lotion.

Creams prescribed by the doctor are often helpful. However, the common treatment of taking the antibiotic, tetracycline, should be discontinued as soon as pregnancy is suspected.

Unusual hair growth does not occur in pregnancy, although light-coloured hair on the skin may become darker and thus noticeable for the first time. The skin tends to become drier in pregnancy and this may produce irritation and minor rashes which can be relieved by moisturising cream or baby oil.

Other changes occurring in the skin are noticed as changes of colour. The nipples darken, and later in pregnancy a thin dark line (linea nigra) appears in the middle of the abdomen. This line will fade after the baby is born. Any abdominal scars may also become pigmented.

Some women notice that their forehead and the skin of their upper and lower jaw also become darker during pregnancy. This condition is called chloasma, or 'the mask of pregnancy'. Unavoidable in those predisposed to it, it is aggravated by exposure to sunlight. If it occurs, take care in the sun and wear a broad-brimmed hat or apply sun block. If you have noticed these changes whilst taking oral contraceptives, they are likely to occur during pregnancy. Chloasma eventually disappears some time after delivery.

Kicks, Hiccups *and* Pulsations

Babies do these things in the second half of the pregnancy. They thump and bump around and appear to have a marvellous time.

Just as their prospective mothers have busy and quiet times, so do they, although these times may not coincide with their mothers' activities. As it is dark inside the uterus, babies do not know when their mums want to go to sleep. Babies are more active after meals, presumably because their increased blood sugar levels give them more energy. Movements are usually felt at 20 to 22 weeks in the first pregnancy and earlier in subsequent pregnancies.

In the last 10 weeks of pregnancy, if the baby does not kick during any one day, you should see your doctor, who may wish to check the baby by listening for its heart-beat with a stethoscope.

Your complexion may darken
▼▼▼

'What's that?'
▼▼▼

BRAXTON-HICKS CONTRACTIONS

The uterus contracts and relaxes all the time whether a woman is pregnant or not. During pregnancy these movements are known as Braxton-Hicks contractions.

As the pregnancy progresses you may notice that these tightenings occur more frequently. They are much more noticeable in a second or third pregnancy than in a first. Sometimes there is a run of tightenings every 15 minutes or so. This is the uterine muscle warming up, just like any good athlete before a race.

When it happens, the best thing to do is to make a cup of tea, put your feet up and sit it out. These contractions differ from those of labour in that they are usually irregular, comparatively painless and without a pattern. Also they are not associated with other signs of labour such as the passage of a mucus plug, bleeding or rupture of the membranes (see Chapter 8: *When should we go to the hospital?*).

There is no reason to sit at home wondering about them. If there is any doubt, contact the hospital or your doctor. You are not expected to know everything about labour, especially if it is your first. Delivery suite staff are experienced and there to help, and nobody minds false alarms.

CONSTIPATION

The bowel is another organ whose function is changed by pregnancy hormones, and as a result constipation and wind almost invariably occur at some time during pregnancy.

Iron tablets can make the situation worse and the doctor may suggest taking them every second day or not at all.

In addition, the uterus pressing on the lower part of the intestine may make elimination difficult, especially in the later part of pregnancy, and may also cause haemorrhoids. If you include extra fibre in your diet you are less likely to suffer from these problems. A high fibre diet is based on food such as bran, prunes, wholegrain bread and cereals, vegetables and salad, nuts, fresh fruit and dried fruits. Also drink plenty of fluids. Emptying the bowel at a regular time each day often helps.

BACKACHE

The back muscles have to work very hard to compensate for the increasing weight up front. As the baby grows and the tummy enlarges, the woman's centre of gravity moves forward and, to balance herself, she must lean back more and more. In addition pregnancy hormones cause ligaments in the pelvis and lower back to soften.

Poor muscle tone can be overcome by regular exercise, and poor posture by making a deliberate effort to stand tall (see Chapter 5: *Is everything alright?*).

The uterus contracts all the time
▼▼▼

'I used to go everyday'
▼▼▼

If backache is really troublesome a maternity corset is very helpful.

Avoid taking analgesics regularly if at all possible. Lifting of heavy loads should be left to someone else, but if absolutely necessary, problems may be averted by squatting before you grasp the load and then lifting by straightening your legs. It is important to keep the back straight while lifting and sitting.

VARICOSE VEINS

A tendency to get varicose veins is usually inherited. During pregnancy the vein walls become softened by the placental hormones oestrogen and progesterone. Then as the uterus enlarges and the pressure in the leg veins increases they swell and may become varicose. Varicose veins are not confined to the legs and may appear in the vulva or around the anus as haemorrhoids. Varicose veins are not to be confused with prominent surface veins in the skin which can be recognised as a fine network of small blue and red vessels.

If you notice you have varicose veins, sitting with your feet up can be most helpful especially when your legs ache. Support stockings or tights can also be very beneficial especially if they are put on first thing in the morning before getting out of bed and starting the day's work.

PILES (HAEMORRHOIDS)

These are varicose veins of the anal canal. They commonly occur towards the end of pregnancy, appearing as small lumps at the edge of the anus. They may itch and occasionally bleed. Avoid constipation by altering your diet. Creams can be given to stop the itch. If haemorrhoids enlarge, suppositories can often reduce their size.

CRAMPS

Most pregnant women get them and they hurt. They may wake in the middle of the night with a sudden and severe muscle spasm.

Why this should occur in late pregnancy is not exactly known but extra salt and calcium in the diet are often found to help.

If cramps persist despite these simple measures a muscle-relaxing drug such as Valium taken before retiring may prevent or diminish attacks. (Valium does not interfere with the development of the baby and, as the cramps occur only intermittently, is not habit-forming.)

Most cramps affect muscles in the calf or in the back of the thigh. When they occur relief can be provided fairly quickly by pressing the back of the leg flat on the bed and having your partner push your foot upwards towards your shin. Laying a hot water-bottle on the muscle helps to relieve cramps and any remaining muscle pain.

TEETH *and* GUMS

Any existing dental problems may deteriorate during pregnancy so a dental check early in pregnancy is wise.

Local anaesthetic in the quantities given for drilling does not harm the baby but always check with your doctor if any antibiotics are suggested.

X-rays are best avoided unless the abdomen is shielded by lead. If the local drinking water supply is not fluoridated fluoride tablets may help to protect mother's and baby's teeth. Remember that by birth a baby's teeth are already formed, though not erupted.

Bleeding from the gums is very common during pregnancy, especially during brushing. In some women the gums will swell and become spongy but they usually return to normal soon after the birth of the baby.

EYES

Seeing spots before the eyes is a common symptom of early pregnancy. However, during late pregnancy if you are carrying a lot of extra fluid or have a headache at the same time, you should check with your hospital or doctor to make sure that high blood pressure is not developing.

ITCHINESS

This may either be confined to the skin of the abdomen or be felt all over the body.

The reasons for these two situations are different. Itchiness of the abdominal skin usually occurs for the first time in late pregnancy and often precedes the appearance of stretch marks.

A more severe itching involving all the skin, including that of the palms and soles, is due to an accumulation of bile salts. If this occurs, medical advice should be sought promptly as mild jaundice may have developed. The diagnosis can be made by blood tests and specific treatment is available. Sometimes the jaundice returns during a subsequent pregnancy or while taking an oral contraceptive.

If itchiness occurs around the vagina, it may be a symptom of thrush, and if it occurs around the anus, it may be due to haemorrhoids or, occasionally, threadworms. All three conditions are readily treatable.

HEARTBURN

The stomach makes acid all the time, and the hormones of pregnancy may allow the gullet (oesophagus) to relax, allowing acid to run back from the stomach. This causes a burning, bilious feeling in the middle of the chest and back of the throat.

This symptom can be relieved in two ways. Firstly, neutralise the acid with either milk or an antacid and, secondly, eat small, frequent meals. Try to avoid making your stomach too full, eat several small meals instead of three big meals, and do not drink fluids during your meals or for half an hour before or afterwards. Sit

Have a dental check early
▼▼▼

Ask about itches
▼▼▼

Small changes in diet often ease heartburn
▼▼▼

up straight and eat food slowly and in a relaxed manner, taking your time between mouthfuls and chewing your food thoroughly. Avoid spicy, fatty or fried foods, and 'windy' foods like onion and cabbage, as these may aggravate the problem.

Try to avoid bending over, and squat or kneel instead. If heartburn is noticed mainly at night, keep your stomach at a lower level than your gullet, either by supporting your shoulders with an extra pillow, or by raising the head-end of the bed on bricks.

Heartburn usually goes away after the baby's head engages or, if this does not happen before labour begins, after the baby is born.

Fluid Retention (Oedema)

It is quite normal for your body to retain extra fluid during pregnancy. This is due to the increased amounts of oestrogen produced by the placenta and baby. The amount of oestrogen produced increases as the pregnancy progresses and so does the amount of fluid retained by the body. In fact, puffy eyes, if not from late nights, are often a give-away to pregnancy.

In most cases the ankles become swollen towards the end of the day because of fluid retention and also from an accumulation of blood in the veins of the legs. This effect is more noticeable during hot weather and is aggravated by standing for prolonged periods.

Puffy ankles are common
▼▼▼

If the swelling extends up over your shins or if the rings on your fingers become tight, you should check with your doctor because you may be developing high blood pressure. This is especially so during the first pregnancy.

When you rest at night the fluid from your legs is taken up and passed as urine. Obviously this results in disturbed nights.

Excess fluid goes away usually within a few days following the baby's birth.

Incontinence

The bladder undergoes many changes during pregnancy. As the uterus enlarges, the bladder stretches because it is attached to the lower part of the front of the uterus. It is because of this change in shape that a woman may occasionally be unable to stop herself passing urine when she coughs, sneezes or even laughs. To try and avoid this you should empty your bladder frequently.

This embarrassing symptom will disappear very soon after the birth of the baby.

Sleeplessness

This often occurs towards the end of pregnancy and is usually because it is hard to find a comfortable position in bed, so the nights are spent tossing and turning.

Some pregnant women feel too tired for sleep and this paradox is not uncommon. Although you may feel dreadful, it does not harm the baby.

If a woman is not working and has no other children to look after she can catch up on her sleep during the day. However, if this is not the first baby, it may occasionally be necessary to take a mild sedative to allow a good night's rest and so break the cycle of sleeplessness. Mild sedatives are not harmful in the last months of pregnancy.

HEADACHES

Tension headaches during pregnancy are quite common, particularly during the early months of pregnancy and on hot days.

Rest, quiet, gentle neck massage, wearing cool, loose clothing and slowing down all help. One or two aspirins or paracetamol occasionally are not harmful, especially if they relax you enough to get some decent rest.

If severe headaches occur during pregnancy you should check with your doctor to see that they are not due to high blood pressure.

LOWER ABDOMINAL PAIN

As the uterus grows out of the pelvis it is not surprising that this large object causes some discomfort. Ligaments may stretch and weight is put on to other organs. The increased weight of the uterus and its tendency to move from side to side may cause groin pains which are often said to resemble a 'stitch'. This pain is made

worse by being overtired, by coughing and by changing position. In most cases it can be relieved by lying curled up on your side.

Not all pain is innocent. If it is severe, or if it continues, and especially if it is associated with bleeding from the vagina, the doctor or hospital must be contacted even in the middle of the night. Maternity hospitals never close. Remember, some women do come into labour much earlier than expected. If there is any doubt, check it out.

RIB PAIN

As the uterus enlarges it pushes up more and more under the ribs. The abdominal muscles attached to the lower ribs stretch, causing the ribs to separate, thereby producing a constant, dull, localised pain. Sitting in a slouched position may allow the ribs to rest on the top of the uterus in late pregnancy; a more erect posture will relieve this discomfort.

A feeling of pressure may be present no matter which way the baby is lying, but it is especially uncomfortable if the baby is presenting as a breech as its head will be up under its mother's ribs (see Chapter 7: *Is there something wrong, doctor?*). Also, some women say that the baby's movements are painful.

Things are much more comfortable when the baby turns around and especially after the baby's head has engaged. Until that time, unfortunately, not a great deal can be done except shift around to find the most comfortable position.

Headaches are common in early pregnancy
▼▼▼

'I can't get comfortable '
▼▼▼

NOSE-BLEEDS (EPISTAXIS)

This is a common problem in pregnancy and is due to an increased blood supply to the nose, probably generated by the pregnancy hormones.

This will usually stop with simple squeezing below the bridge of the nose for five to 10 minutes.

Nose-bleeds are common
▼▼▼

NERVE PAINS

Pain in the hand(s) may be caused by pressure on the main nerve to the hand as it passes through a tunnel in tissue in the wrist (carpel tunnel syndrome). This usually occurs late in pregnancy and is due to swelling of the tissue following increased fluid retention. It is usually worst in the early hours of the morning and in addition there is stiffness of the finger joints which may take an hour or two to disappear after waking. This condition will disappear sometime after delivery. Temporary relief can usually be obtained by wearing special wrist splints at night. In severe cases cortisone injections may provide relief.

A strange type of pain on the foot and side of the thigh is caused by irritation of a nerve passing under a ligament in the groin. This is also due to fluid retention and usually disappears completely after delivery.

Pain in the buttock and down the back of the leg (sciatica) is rarely due to spinal prolems during pregnancy, unless they are pre-existing. It is a reaonably common symptom and mostly due to pressure on nerves in the pelvis by the baby during the second half of pregnancy.

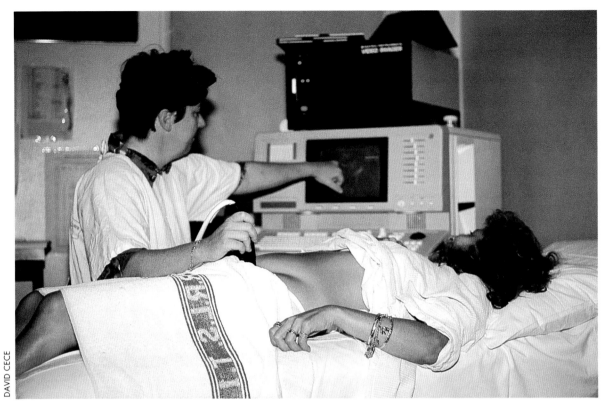

An ultrasonic examination is a simple, non-invasive test which provides an image of the fetus. It is used to measure the size of the fetus and monitor its growth rate.

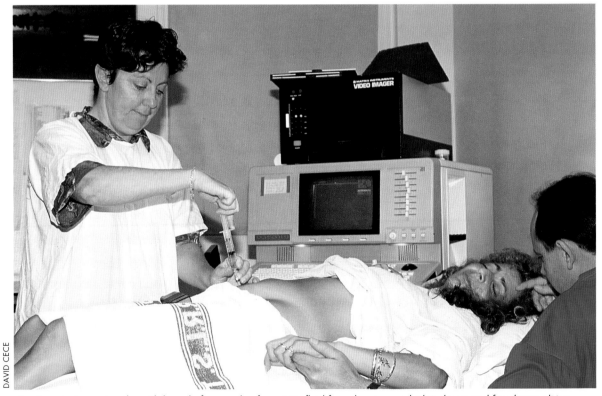

Amniocentesis requires the withdrawal of a sample of amniotic fluid from the uterus, which is then tested for abnormalities.

DAVID CECE

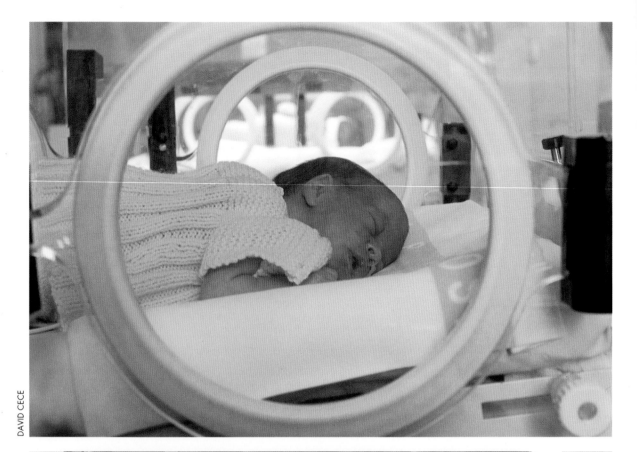

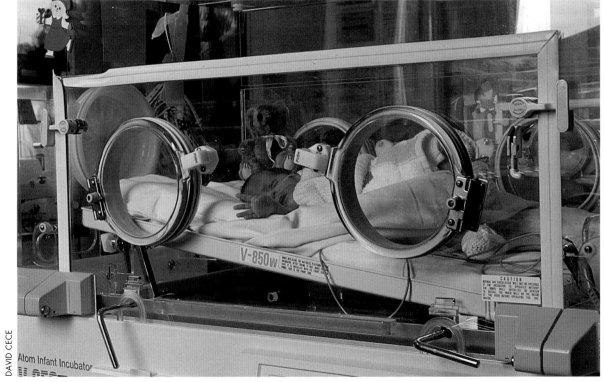

Top and above: A pre-term baby may need to be nursed in a humidicrib.

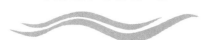

CHAPTER 5

IS EVERY-THING ALL RIGHT?

Prenatal Care

Modern prenatal care was pioneered by a Scotsman, John Ballantyne, in the early years of this century. Since then, prenatal care has made such an enormous contribution to pregnancy and childbirth that few people in Australia today have experienced a relative or friend dying as a result of pregnancy. Significant contributions have also come from improved social conditions, blood transfusion, antibiotics and management of labour.

The Royal Hospital for Women, Paddington opened its Antenatal Clinic in August 1912, the third in the world. It is also the hospital holding the record for the longest continuous service to pregnant women in the British Commonwealth.

Early care allows for the best outcome

▼▼▼

Prenatal care can be divided into two broad areas: education and supervision.

Education is concerned with dietary needs and with physical and psychological preparation for pregnancy and childbirth.

The aim of supervision is to detect variations from normal and, where applicable, commence treatment. Although a lot of problems related to pregnancy do not appear to be preventable, early detection often improves the outcome for both mother and baby.

In Australia the person best qualified to play a supervisory role during pregnancy is a medical practitioner.

WHEN *to* SEE *the* DOCTOR

Symptoms of early pregnancy have been described in Chapter 4: ...*and this?* However their occurrence is not the signal to rush off for confirmation of pregnancy. It is better to wait until the second period is missed, unless nausea is unduly severe or bleeding occurs, as a more accurate assessment of the pregnancy can be made at that stage. However with the current bed shortages in obstetric hospitals an early pregnancy test is important to ensure the hospital of your choice.

WHICH DOCTOR *to* SEE

The majority of women consult their family doctor for confirmation of pregnancy. Few family doctors outside country areas offer obstetric care these days and so the majority of women are referred to an obstetrician to supervise their pregnancy and labour. A lot of women prefer to be looked after by an obstetrician who has attended their friends or relatives or who has access to a particular hospital. Almost without exception such requests for referral are met without demur.

It may happen that a rapport does not develop between the woman and the doctor to whom she has been referred. This is usually apparent at an early stage and it is at this time that she should request transfer to the care of a person whom she feels will be more suited to herself.

Most women prefer to give birth in hospitals
▼▼▼

You can choose your doctor
▼▼▼

WHERE *to* HAVE *the* BABY

The overwhelming majority of women prefer to give birth in a hospital where specialist help is immediately available for both mother and baby if the need arises. Not all women like the atmosphere of a hospital, and some consumer groups have reacted against the use of technological advances in obstetrics that have developed in the 1970s and 1980s. There has been a demand for non-intervention obstetrics, the so-called 'natural birth', and a belief that obstetricians interfere too much with this natural process.

There is no such thing as a 'no risk' pregnancy only a 'low risk' pregnancy, and even with this group complications can occur with frightening rapidity. Most obstetric units have relaxed the rigid routines of yesteryear, and made architectural changes to create a more home-like atmosphere in the labour suite.

The development of Birth Centres attached to obstetric hospitals has gone further. Here, carefully selected patients are seen by midwives who are closely involved with their prenatal care, and education, and who develop a trusting relationship with the patient, her partner, other children of the couple, and other support persons. The philosophy of the Birth Centre is to allow the labour to progress, with no interference, to a normal delivery, but still under very careful supervision. Any departure from a normal labour allows the patient to be transferred to the hospital delivery suite for further treatment.

This type of arrangement is very popular with a proportion of the community, and the number of such Birth Centres has increased. They are expensive for hospitals to run because of the one-to-one staffing, and could never fully replace the modern obstetric delivery suite.

However, there is an enormous amount of satisfaction to those women who successfully deliver their babies surrounded by their family and friends, and the centres provide a very safe alternative to the potentially more hazardous experience of home birth.

OTHER CHILDREN PRESENT AT DELIVERY

Most hospital labour wards are not equipped to cope with other children being present at the delivery. Of course places like Birth Centres are ideally set up for these. Because the father is busy supporting and encouraging the mother-to-be, then it is vital that a third adult support person trusted by both and particularly by the children is present in the delivery room. Children under four do not seem to get much benefit from watching a birth. It is necessary for the midwife or obstetrician to feel very comfortable with children being present and to know the child beforehand. It must always be the child's decision whether he or she wishes to attend in the first place and at all times that child must be given the option of retiring should they become bored, distressed, tired or hungry. Children that are coerced into staying get little enjoyment or memorable experience from the birth and often will go into a corner and watch the television, play with their toys or simply go to sleep. Those that feel very positive about the birth will come over and touch the pregnant tummy, help listen to the baby's heart beat, make positive and encouraging noises, gently help and rub tired backs with oil, do special favours such as wiping their mother's face with a face cloth. Somehow they seem to see beyond the pain, mess and distress and have a wonderful broad vision of the wider aspects of the joy of birthing. If the children are carefully guided and educated beforehand it is exceedingly rare for that child to end up being disturbed or distressed. In fact just the opposite is the case where most children feel very warm and loving, having been there to meet and greet their sister or brother and this loving spiritual bond seems to continue.

Children can enjoy watching the birth
▼▼▼

THE FIRST PRENATAL VISIT

This is by far the most important visit during a woman's pregnancy. It is the time when her recollection of important recent events is clearest — for example, she can remember the date of her last period, whether she has had any bleeding since then, whether she has taken any tablets since her last period. It is therefore the best time for the doctor to gather a full history from the patient. Things that seem insignificant may have a bearing on the outcome of the pregnancy.

The first visit consists of an interview, a physical examination and various investigations (tests).

The first visit is most important
▼▼▼

INTERVIEW

Initially this concentrates on the current pregnancy. When was the first day of the last period, and were periods regular? If the day of conception is known, it is invaluable information. What form of contraception has been used and when did it stop? (Where amenorrhoea has continued after stopping taking the Pill, the time conception took place is often difficult to determine.) All this information enables the doctor to estimate the likely date of the baby's arrival.

The doctor will need to know about all previous pregnancies, even if they ended in miscarriage or abortion, and will also ask when each pregnancy occurred and how long it lasted. Was the pregnancy normal and how did labour start? How long did labour last? What method of delivery was used? Did the placenta separate normally, were stitches needed to repair a vaginal tear, was an episiotomy performed (see Chapter 10: *Is it alright if I push?*)? What was the weight and sex of the baby and did it have any problems after birth? Was the baby breastfed or bottle fed?

The reason for all these questions is that some situations may be recurrent, such as pre-term labour, small babies and bleeding associated with the failure of the placenta to separate properly.

If a previous baby has been delivered by caesarean section it is unwise to consider giving birth either in a birth cenre or at home. However most women can have a vaginal birth following caesarean section. If more than one child has been born by caesarean section most obstetricians would not recommend a subsequent labour.

General information is also important: age (mainly because the incidence of some congenital abnormalities increases over the age of 35) drug allergies, any history of blood transfusion, smoking habits, if any, and alcohol consumption. Usual weight is noted, to serve as a point of comparison for weight gain during the pregnancy. It is important to know how tall you are and how heavy you were when you were born, as it will give the doctor some idea of how big the baby is likely to be. Information about your job or profession and that of your partner is helpful to the doctor to complete the picture of you as a person.

Family history is also important. Some illnesses tend to run in families and two of these, hypertension and diabetes, may be unmasked by pregnancy. Some congenital defects tend to be recurrent and some of these can be detected early in pregnancy. Sometimes difficulties during pregnancy tend to recur in families, so the doctor will want to know something of your mother's (and sisters') obstetric history. Did they have hypertension, small babies, caesarean sections?

A history of twins is also important. The ability to have non-identical twins is thought to be handed down through female members of the family. However, this is not usually the case with identical twins.

PHYSICAL EXAMINATION

This is a full physical examination as it is important to exclude the possibility of serious disease, to check that the breasts and nipples are normal and that you are generally fit.

Height, weight and blood pressure are measured and then the heart, lungs, breasts and neck are examined. Then the abdomen, arms and legs are checked.

Next, a careful internal pelvic examination allows the doctor to check the size of the uterus and relate this to the date of the last period. Sometimes a discrepancy between the two is noted, and this can be checked by an ultrasonic examination. Occasionally, an ovarian cyst may be found which could be large enough to interfere with normal labour. If one is discovered, it should be checked at intervals and, if still present at 14 to 15 weeks, should be removed. The reason for waiting is that most cysts will have disappeared by 14 weeks.

It is not usual to try and assess the size of the pelvis at this visit, as this is better done in the last month of pregnancy, if there is any doubt that pelvic size may not be adequate.

TESTS

A sample of urine is tested for sugar and protein. This is important as the presence of sugar may indicate a tendency to diabetes, and protein may mean a bladder infection or, rarely, some kidney disease.

Some blood tests are essential in early pregnancy. Some which may have been performed before will not be repeated, for example blood group and German measles (rubella) antibody level.

BLOOD COUNT

This will tell if there is anaemia and it will give a guide to the type of anaemia. A haemoglobin level of average or above average means that no iron supplement is required provided the diet is adequate.

BLOOD GROUPING

This is done early in the pregnancy in order to avoid the possibility of having to do it in an emergency later on. It will also show if the Rhesus (Rh) factor is positive or negative. If you are Rhesus negative, additional blood tests will need to be performed later in the pregnancy to look for antibodies.

BLOOD GROUP ANTIBODIES

All women, whether Rhesus negative or positive, need a blood group antibody screen at the commencement of each pregnancy. Any antibodies will usually have been formed during a previous pregnancy or as a result of a blood transfusion. Some of these antibodies can cross the placenta to the baby, causing it to become anaemic, while others cause problems if blood has to be crossmatched later should a transfusion should be necessary.

Screening for blood group antibodies will be repeated at 28 weeks, and again between 34 and 36 weeks for women who are Rhesus negative, as some antibodies may appear for the first time later in pregnancy.

Routine tests are important
▼▼▼

All women need a blood group antibody test
▼▼▼

RUBELLA IMMUNITY

The majority of women are immune to German measles (rubella) because they have been either infected by the virus or immunised. If an antibody level has not been estimated previously it will be done now, as not all immunisations produce immunity. Women whose antibody levels show that they are immune will be reassured and those who are not immune will be provided with a baseline against which later comparisons can be made, if necessary.

If a woman develops a rash during pregnancy, another rubella antibody level test can be performed two weeks after the rash appears and the two results compared. If the antibody level rises twofold it means that the rash was due to German measles and if this occurred in the first three months of pregnancy there is a danger of congenital malformation. In such instances the parents may request that the pregnancy be terminated.

VDRL

Named after the Venereal Diseases Research Laboratory, this is a screening test for syphilis. Untreated syphilis in the mother can lead to congenital infection of the baby. Fortunately, maternal infection is readily curable with antibiotics. Syphilis is not a common disease and some doctors do not perform the test. However, the VDRL is a simple and cheap test, and early treatment will prevent the possibility of malformation in the child.

Non-venereal infections can give a positive result (false positive), so when a positive result is obtained, further blood tests will show if the result is really due to syphilis.

ALPHA-FETO-PROTEIN (AFP)

This substance makes its way into the mother's blood from the baby. Raised levels may be found if the baby has abnormalities such as anencephaly or spina bifida and some other rarer congenital abnormalities. However, the test does not detect all babies with these abnormalities (false negative result) and it may be abnormally high in other situations which may be absolutely normal (false positive result). High levels of AFP in the mother's blood require the testing of an additional blood sample. If the level is still high, an ultrasound examination can be performed to check the baby's size and to see if its structure is normal. A multiple pregnancy may be found. In addition, an amniocentesis will provide a sample of amniotic fluid in which the AFP level can then be determined. If this level is normal, the presence of severe forms of spina bifida can be eliminated.

As with the VDRL, doctors are not always in agreement about the usefulness of this test in Australia as the number of babies born with spina bifida and anencephaly is lower here than in most other countries where data is available.

'Did my rubella injection protect me?'

▼▼▼

BACILLURIA SCREENING TEST (BST)

This test, performed on a clean midstream sample of urine, picks up otherwise undetectable kidney and bladder infections. About 6 per cent of pregnant women have a urinary infection and are not aware of it because they have no symptoms. These infections are important because at least one third of them may develop into a serious kidney infection (pyelonephritis) as the pregnancy progresses.

Early treatment is safe for both mother and baby and will eliminate this risk.

Again, not all doctors perform this test or only do so if there is a past history of kidney or bladder infection.

HEPATITIS B

Hepatitis B is a very contagious disease which can have serious longterm side effects. If the mother tests positive there is no effect on the baby during pregnancy; however the baby should be immunised against this disease and this should commence shortly after birth. Because the disease is highly contagious, patients who test positive are barrier nursed in hospital.

PLASMA GLUCOSE

This test may be used to see if a woman has developed diabetes during her pregnancy (see conditions which may be aggravated by pregnancy).

The test is offered to all patients by some obstetricians and to those women considered most likely to develop gestational diabetes by others. Women most at risk are those over 35 years of age, those who are overweight, having had a baby previously who weighed 4.5 kg (10 lb) or more and women who have more than one close relative with diabetes.

The test should be performed between 28 to 32 weeks. Like some other tests there is no uniform agreement about the type of test to be used or what levels should be regarded as abnormal.

TRIPLE SCREEN (DOWN'S SYNDROME TEST)

Recently this test has been introduced to detect Down's Syndrome in women under 35 years of age who are usually considered as having a low risk of bearing a child with this disorder. The test involves the measurement of three different hormones in a sample of blood taken when a woman is 16 to 18 weeks pregnant and assesses a woman's risk as either low, moderate or high for having a baby with Down's Syndrome. However, the test has proved to be less valuable in practice than hoped as it has high false positive and false negative results and any test which judges a woman to be at high risk has to be investigated in mid pregnancy by either amniocentesis, placental biopsy or fetal blood sampling. Fortunately most of these tests show the baby to have normal chromosomes. The Triple Screen test doubles the detection rate of Down's Syndrome from 30 to 60 per cent.

Women under 35 are tested for Down's Syndrome too

▼▼▼

HIV TESTING

There is no clear recommendation regarding this. The test should, like all other tests, only be performed with the patient's consent. Some doctors screen all women whilst others screen only those regarded as having a high risk of becoming exposed to the virus. These include past or present IV drug users, women with bisexual partners, those with HIV positive partners, sex industry workers and women who received blood transfusions before 1984. If positive, the woman may elect to have the pregnancy terminated although the risk of the baby becoming infected is probably as low as 12–15 per cent.

During labour patients will be barrier nursed, however there is no need for isolation from other patients either before or after giving birth.

GROUP B STREPTOCOCCUS SCREENING

Group B Streptococcus is a bacterium which lives in the vagina of about 5 per cent of women at some time or another. If present during labour it may cause a severe or even fatal infection in a small proportion of babies whose mothers are carrying the bacteria at that time. Some doctors screen all women for this organism, usually between 26 to 32 weeks by vaginal swabbing, and if it is found to be present prescribe antibiotics, usually a penicillin type, for the woman during labour as this is known to lessen the chances of severe infection. Ideally the drug is given intravenously before the membranes rupture. However, nature

is fickle; the organism may disappear after it is found or appear for the first time after the swab has been taken, or the membrances can rupture either before the onset of labour or admission to hospital.

CERVICAL SMEAR (PAP TEST)

If a smear has not been done in the last one or two years, most doctors will take this opportunity to inspect the cervix and take a smear from it. Other doctors prefer to wait until after the baby is born to take a smear.

ULTRASONIC EXAMINATION

This is a test which involves the use of sound waves to build up a picture (see Chapter 6: *Everybody tells me something different*). It is harmless to both mother and baby. It may be used to confirm that a patient is pregnant, measure the size of the baby and see if there is more than one baby. This is a most useful test if there is doubt about what is really happening and if a problem such as bleeding occurs. However, it has never been shown that an ultrasonic examination during every pregnancy significantly alters the outcome for mothers or babies. Routine use of ultrasound would significantly alter the size of the health budget as it is an expensive procedure. Ultrasonic examinations cannot totally exclude the possibility of fetal abnormality.

Some doctors believe that every woman should have an ultrasound examination at least once during pregnancy. The time mostly recommended for this to occur is between 18 to 20 weeks because this

'But all my friends have had a scan'
▼▼▼

is the time one can best see the baby's structure.

At this stage, you and your doctor should have reached a point of mutual ease and confidence where discussion can take place about hospital facilities, attitudes to pregnancy and labour, breastfeeding and circumcision.

This is the time to decide whether to stick with each other. Do not wait until two weeks before the baby is due. Ask if the doctor has holidays scheduled when the baby is due. Some will know, others will not. Hopefully most can tell well in advance if their plans change. Even so, most doctors have a weekend off or go out at night and some even get sick! So it is possible they may not be there at the birth. However, most doctors are present at the delivery of the majority of their patients.

SUBSEQUENT VISITS

After the first visit, further visits are needed during the pregnancy for two reasons.

Firstly, you and your doctor get to know each other better and secondly, the progress of the pregnancy can be checked. Each visit consists of a conversation about you and your pregnancy. If between visits you think of questions to ask, make a note of them so that they are not overlooked.

At these visits weight and blood pressure are checked. An abdominal examination will establish the size of the uterus and a sample of urine will be tested for sugar and protein. These tests can help to detect some

problems early, and serious complications may therefore be avoided. These problems include:

1 Hypertension. If unchecked, this may lead to pre-eclampsia or antepartum haemorrhage (see Chapter 7: *Is there something wrong, doctor?*). It can be detected by checking the blood pressure and by urine tests.

2 Small babies (growth retardation). This is detected by failure of the mother to gain weight and by the uterus not growing properly.

3 Multiple pregnancy. The uterus is obviously too large for the stage of pregnancy.

4 Breech presentation. This situation is important towards the end of pregnancy and is detected by feeling the baby's head at the top of the uterus rather than in its more usual situation at the bottom.

5 Bleeding. This is unavoidable and unpreventable, but is fortunately uncommon.

6 Pre-term labour. Only one cause of pre-term labour is avoidable. This is when the labour is due to cervical incompetence (see Chapter 7: *Is there something wrong, doctor?*).

FREQUENCY OF VISITS

How often visits should take place depends on the patient and her doctor. For instance, a woman having her first baby needs to be seen at intervals of four to six weeks up to 26 weeks, then every two to three weeks till 36 weeks, and then each week until the baby is born.

Problems may occur, so regular visits are important
▼ ▼ ▼

The reason for this type of timing is best understood when you know about the problems that can be anticipated. Most multiple pregnancies become obvious between 20 and 28 weeks. Hypertension mostly develops after 28 weeks but is most frequently seen from 34 weeks onwards. A breech presentation that is likely to persist is diagnosed during the last four weeks.

Many doctors perform a vaginal examination to assess pelvic size in the last two or three weeks of pregnancy.

If the pregnancy continues past the due date, frequent visits enable a close watch to be kept on the health of the mother and baby.

A history of uncomplicated pregnancies is taken into account: the earlier visits are usually at six weekly intervals until 28 weeks, three weekly until 37 weeks and then weekly until the baby is born.

Of course there may be variations from these two examples. Sometimes visits need to be more frequent, especially if the mother has a special problem, for example a pre-existing illness such as diabetes. If problems have appeared in a previous pregnancy, a closer watch than usual is needed during the current pregnancy.

'Can I play squash?'

▼▼▼

COURTESY CARD

Most doctors and hospitals provide women with a duplicate copy of their prenatal history, commonly known as a courtesy card. This is filled in at each prenatal visit and should be carried by the woman at all times. The information on this card does away with a lot of unnecessary questions during admission to hospital. Should the mother be admitted in an emergency to a different hospital, this card is invaluable and saves much time and effort. It may even save lives.

LIFESTYLE

EXERCISE

It is important to remain fit during pregnancy and this is best done by continuing to participate in your usual sporting activities. Regular exercise, especially walking or swimming, will help improve muscle tone and general well-being. Towards the end of pregnancy ligaments soften and muscles become stretched, so avoid violent activity and heavy lifting.

WORK

The tiredness experienced during early pregnancy usually lessens during the middle part and most women in their first pregnancy are able to work till 32 or 34 weeks without becoming unduly tired. However, it is common for women to say after they have left work, 'I didn't realise how tired I was. This is such a common remark that it would seem wise to leave full-time work six to eight weeks before the baby is due. This decision depends of course on your type of work, age and general health. Sometimes pregnancy complications have to be considered as well.

A woman who already has children often has no choice but to keep on working up to the time she goes into hospital.

With the first pregnancy, the few weeks before the baby comes will be the last time parents can relax together for quite a while. Make the most of it.

REST

The amount of rest a woman requires during pregnancy varies. Fatigue demands rest. Most pregnant women feel they require more sleep at night. As the pregnancy advances, it is more comfortable to rest or sleep on your side. This position also benefits the baby as it improves the blood supply to the uterus and therefore the placenta. A rest during the day is beneficial.

DRUGS

Where possible, drugs should be avoided during pregnancy and smoking stopped.

Similarly, alcohol consumption should be limited. Fortunately, for a lot of women this is easy, as alcohol intolerance is not an uncommon symptom of pregnancy. However, an occasional drink before dinner or a glass of wine with it have not been shown to have any detrimental effects on the fetus. Untoward effects on the baby ascribed to alcohol have so far only been recorded in women who have been heavy drinkers.

Excessive coffee drinking and hence high caffeine intake should be avoided during pregnancy as babies whose mother drink many cups of coffee are thought to have withdrawal symptoms in the first one or two weeks after birth.

The use of drugs such as heroin and methadone by mothers can produce severe problems for the fetus. Almost always these babies do not grow to their full potential and frequently they are born early because of premature labour. In addition the babies often suffer severely in the newborn period because of symptoms of drug withdrawal. Neither heroin, methadone nor drugs such as marijuana have been shown to cause fetal structural abnormality.

Cocaine should not be taken at any time during pregnancy as it causes blood vessels to constrict and so less blood gets to the uterus and therefore the baby and placenta. Cocaine may also cause bleeding from behind the placenta later in pregnancy which can be severe enough to be fatal to the baby.

Where constant medication is required, for example asthma or epilepsy, the advice of an obstetrician should be sought as soon as possible.

Occasionally an illness such as bronchitis or a kidney infection occurs during the course of a pregnancy, requiring treatment with antibiotics. With the exception of tetracyclines, all the commonly available antibiotics which can be taken as either tablets or capsules are safe.

Put your feet up
▼▼▼

Stop smoking!
▼▼▼

Avoid excessive coffee drinking
▼▼▼

SEXUAL ACTIVITY

Sexual activity need not be restricted because of pregnancy. However, a woman's sexual desire may increase or diminish. Except in a few cases, intercourse is possible until the end of pregnancy. However, variations in position will be necessary as the woman's abdomen becomes larger.

Towards the end of pregnancy, especially if the baby's head is engaged, there is very little room in the woman's vagina to accommodate her partner's penis, but a little ingenuity goes a long way. Sometimes intercourse results in a slightly bloodstained discharge from the vagina. This is usually not a cause for alarm as the cervix becomes very soft in pregnancy and can bleed on touching.

Some doctors advise against intercourse during the last two months of pregnancy because semen contains substances called prostaglandins that theoretically can produce uterine contractions and therefore cause pre-term labour. Whilst this rule is not observed universally, it would be wise for a woman who has previously had a pre-term labour to abstain from intercourse for the last two months of pregnancy unless a condom is used.

If there has been bleeding during the pregnancy, ask your doctor if intercourse is likely to cause problems. If the bleeding is due to placenta praevia, intercourse should cease forthwith (see Chapter 7: *Is there something wrong, doctor?*).

TRAVEL

Air travel is possible up to 28 weeks without any queries from airlines. From 28 to 34 weeks a doctor's certificate of fitness to travel is essential, and after 34 weeks most air travel is restricted.

Finally, it is sensible to carry a doctor's certificate if travelling overseas.

PROBLEMS WITH YOUR UNDER-THREE-YEAR-OLD WHILE YOU ARE PREGNANT

The child at home while mother is pregnant will join in when everybody starts getting excited about a new baby coming. Any child is likely to show symptoms of anxiety as the mother slows up, changes shape, and does strange things (by the child's standards) in the later months of pregnancy. This may involve changes in behaviour, such as increased whingeing and clinging, poor sleep patterns, loss of appetite or increased demand for parental attention. In the later months of pregnancy, mothers often start feeling guilty that they are not devoting enough time to the older child and they tend to sit and play with them more, whereas they should push the child into more independent activity, so that the child will be less demanding.

Arrangements should be made for the child to stay with, or have familiar people stay with the child, so that there is no rude shock when the mother goes to hospital. If mother leaves to go to hospital during the night, she must wake the child to say 'goodbye', otherwise the child is

Try different positions

▼▼▼

Other children may feel anxious

▼▼▼

likely to wake every night for the next six months to make sure that mother is still at home.

The under-three-year-old does not understand how mother can be a mother to more than one child, whereas the over-three-year-old can fully understand that mummy can be mother to several. For the under-three-year-old it is most important to get used to seeing mother cuddling babies to realise that this is not a challenge to his or her relationship with mother.

PREPARATION *for* BREASTFEEDING

This commences at the first prenatal visit, when the doctor will check the woman's breasts and nipples.

If the nipples are inverted it does not necessarily mean that she will not be able to breastfeed, because if the nipple becomes erect either when stimulated or when exposed to cold, it will almost certainly evert when the time comes to breastfeed. If this does not occur, discussion with a midwife or a lactation consultant can be beneficial.

Becoming familiar with your breasts during the pregnancy by handling them and using them in love making (if you and your partner find this comfortable) is the best preparation for breastfeeding. Ointments and creams are unnecessary as they alter the natural flora of the skin. Fresh air, a little sunshine and normal hygiene will keep the area healthy. Routine expression is unnecessary.

NUTRITION DURING PREGNANCY

Good nutrition is fundamental to the development of a strong, healthy baby. The dietary preparation for your pregnancy began with the eating pattern established way back in your childhood. A lifetime of healthy eating ensures that you enter your pregnancy in the best of nutritional health. Also, some diseases such as spina bifida have been linked to a dietary deficiency. In the case of spina bifida, studies have shown that taking folates in the early stages of pregnancy dramatically reduce the chances of neural tube defects. Foods rich in folates are vegetables, fruit, legumes, wholegrain breads and cereals.

Just as your mother's nutritional habits influenced your way of eating, so yours will in turn influence those of your children and consequently their nutritional health.

When you are pregnant it is important to eat wisely, as this is the time when your needs for nutrients are increased by the demands of the growing baby. You will need to eat good, nutritious food from the earliest weeks of the pregnancy to provide the necessary minerals and vitamins.

The best diet to follow when you are pregnant is one containing a variety of foods chosen from the major food groups.

It is important to eat three good meals each day. Missing meals means that you and your baby miss out on needed energy and nutrients for a time, and is not recommended.

Help breastfeeding get off to a good start
▼▼▼

A healthy diet is very important
▼▼▼

FOOD GROUP	SUGGESTED DAILY INTAKE	COMMENTS
Bread and cereal	4 servings or more 1 serving is: 1 slice of bread, or ½ cup cooked rice, spaghetti, macaroni, noodles, rolled oats, or ¾ cup breakfast cereal, or 2 crispbread	These foods provide energy, protein, vitamins (especially B vitamins) and minerals. Wholegrain breads and cereals are preferable as they contain more fibre and nutrients. Crispbread may occasionally be substituted for bread to provide variety in the diet.

Fruit and fruit juice, vegetables and salad	4 servings or more
	Include 1 vitamin C fruit or vegetable daily:
	  citrus fruit, berry fruit, raw tomatoes, raw capsicum, fresh pineapple, mango, rockmelon, pawpaw, Brussels sprouts, broccoli and juices from these fruits.
	Include green vegetables daily.
	Include yellow vegetables and fruits regularly:
	  carrots, pumpkin, apricots, rockmelon, pawpaw.
		These foods are major sources of vitamins (especially vitamin C, folic acid and Vitamin A), minerals and fibre in your diet.
		
		Choose pure fruit juices, not fruit juice drinks or cordials.
		
		Fresh fruits are preferable to canned or stewed fruit.
		
		Vegetables should be cooked in a small amount of water until they are just cooked. Do not add bicarbonate of soda to vegetables as this destroys the vitamins.

Milk and milk products	600 to 900 ml Note: Teenage pregnancy 900 ml 30 g hard cheese = 200 ml milk 200 g yoghurt = 250 ml milk	These foods are high in calcium, which is essential for bone and teeth formation, protein, which is used to build muscles and new tissues, and vitamins (especially vitamin A and riboflavin). Note: Cream cheese, cottage cheese and ricotta are low in calcium and are not suitable substitutes for milk. Milk may be used in tea or coffee, as a drink, flavoured, on cereal, in desserts, soups or sauces. Low fat milk, skim milk and low fat yoghurt may be used instead of full cream milk and yoghurt.
Meat, poultry, fish, eggs, cheese and legumes	2 to 3 servings. Include one of these foods at 2 or 3 of your meals each day. 1 average serving is: 75–100 g meat, fish, poultry, cheese, or 1 to 2 eggs, or ½ cup cooked legumes	These foods contain protein, energy and many vitamins and minerals. Meat, chicken and fish are major dietary sources of iron, used to form new blood cells.
Butter, margarine, and other fats and oils	Use in moderation.	These foods are very high in energy (kilojoules). Butter and table margarine are rich sources of vitamins A and D.
Water	6 to 8 glasses or more	Found in milk, soup, fruit juice and other drinks. Water is necessary for efficient kidney function and bowel and function.

Construct your meals carefully and include protein foods, bread and cereals, and fresh fruit or vegetables at each meal.

SUGGESTED MEAL PATTERN

Breakfast
Cereal
Egg, cheese or meat if wanted
Toast or bread with butter or table margarine
Milk
Tea or coffee if wanted

Light meal
Meat, poultry, fish, eggs, cheese or legumes
Salad or cooked vegetables
Bread with butter or table margarine
Fresh fruit
Milk or yoghurt
Tea or coffee if wanted

Main meal
Meat, poultry, fish, eggs, cheese or legumes
Potato, rice, pasta or bread with butter or table margarine
Other vegetables or salad
Fresh fruit
Milk or milk pudding
Tea or coffee if wanted

Between meals
Have fruit or milk between meals or if you are very hungry, have plain biscuits with cheese, nuts, dried fruit or yoghurt.

It is not wise to eat snacks between meals, especially if you are putting on too much weight. However, if you are hungry choose one of the nutritious foods listed above. Avoid eating sweet foods such as cakes and sweet biscuits.

If you are eating a nutritious diet such as the one described, you will not need extra vitamin or mineral supplements, with the possible exceptions of iron, folic acid and fluoride, which may be recommended by your doctor.

The amount of iron in the diet can be raised by increasing your intake of iron-rich foods such as liver and liver products (for example, pâté), kidney, red meat, chicken, fish and oysters. Cereals, green leafy vegetables, eggs and legumes also supply iron but it is not as easily absorbed.

If you eat a piece of fruit containing vitamin C, such as an orange or orange juice, at the same meal as these iron-containing foods you will absorb more of the iron.

It is not a good idea to drink much coffee or other beverages containing caffeine such as tea, cola and cocoa. Limit these drinks to two to three cups or glasses per day. Excessive alcohol is harmful to the unborn baby. However a glass of wine before or with the evening meal causes no problems.

RECOMMENDED WEIGHT GAIN

You do not need to 'eat for two' when you are pregnant. The extra milk provided in the suggested daily intake is probably all the extra food that you require.

The average weight gain for pregnancy is 10 to 13 kg. An adequate gain can be achieved by eating a nourishing, well balanced diet. It is important to gain weight during pregnancy. If you are overweight or

Eat wisely
▼▼▼

Don't eat snacks
▼▼▼

you have gained too much weight, do not use severe reduction diets as this may affect the baby's growth as well as reduce your intake of vitally needed nutrients. Diets with less than 6300 kilojoules (1500 calories) are particularly undesirable. If you are underweight when you become pregnant it is advisable to aim at a weight gain of at least 13 to 14 kg during your pregnancy.

A steady weight gain is desirable. Aim to put on about 1 to 2 kg during your first three months, and from then on about 1 to 2 kg each month.

Certain foods are high in kilojoules and low in nutritional value, and it is wise to restrict your consumption of these foods, especially if you are putting on too much weight. Such foods include sugar and sweets, chocolates, soft drinks, cordials, biscuits, cakes, honey and jams, as well as fried and fatty foods such as oil, meat pies,

sausage rolls, spring rolls, chips and other snack foods.

It is not necessary to restrict your salt intake unless your doctor advises you to do so, but this is unlikely.

PREGNANT TEENAGER

Teenagers, especially those under 17, need to eat well because their own bodies are still growing. They will need to increase their food intake to meet both their own growth requirements as well as those of the baby. In addition to the diet already outlined, 900 ml or more of milk should be taken each day, as well as extra protein foods, fruits and vegetables, breads and cereals. You may also need nutritious snacks between meals. Do not restrict your food intake or skip meals or follow a weight loss diet while you are pregnant. It is important to gain weight while you are expecting a baby.

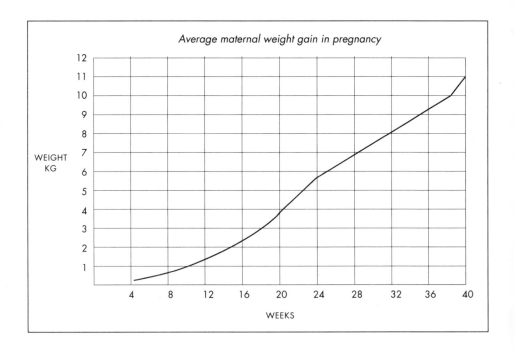

Average maternal weight gain in pregnancy

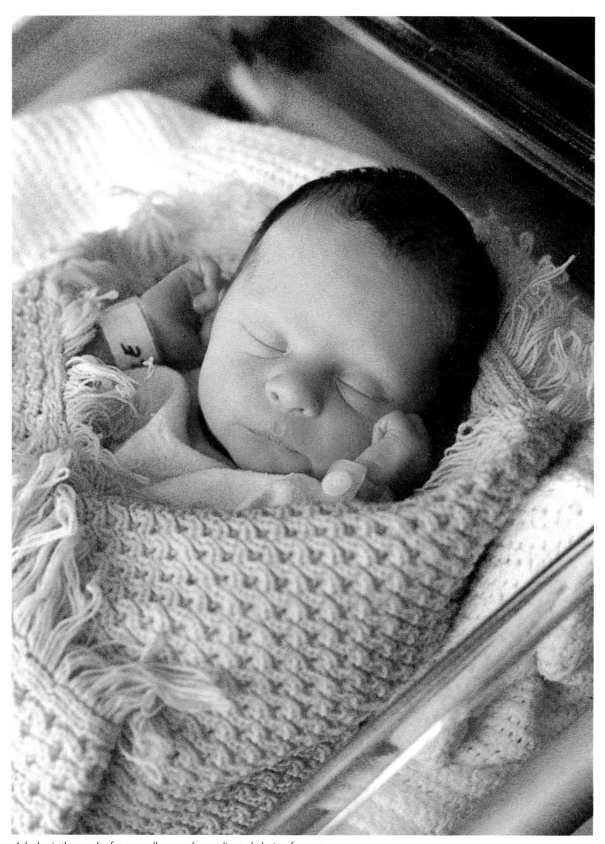

A baby is the result of a marvellous and complicated chain of events.

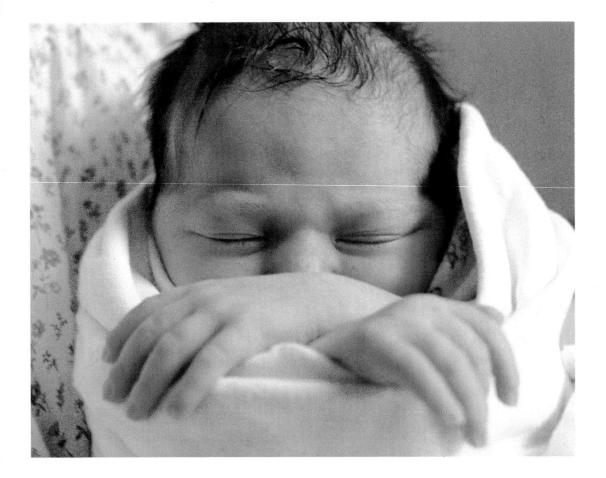

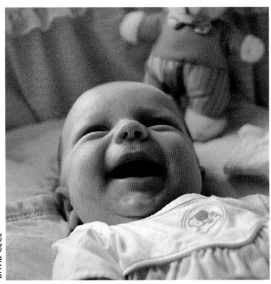

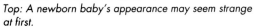

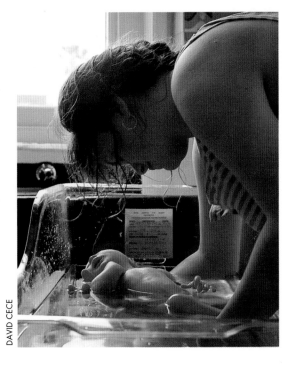

Top: A newborn baby's appearance may seem strange at first.

Above: Babies don't cry all the time!

Right: Babies may hate to be bathed in the first weeks of life — make sure you talk to and reassure your baby while dressing, undressing and bathing him or her.

PREGNANT VEGETARIAN

If you eat a variety of foods from the major food groups previously outlined you can easily plan a nutritionally sound vegetarian diet. You need to ensure an adequate intake of energy, protein and iron. Protein foods such as cow's milk, goat's milk, soy milk, yoghurt, eggs, cheese, legumes, nuts, seeds and fish should be included regularly in your diet, and you may need to eat extra bread and cereal foods.

If you are a total vegetarian (vegan) and do not eat any animal foods at all, you will need a vitamin B12 supplement as adequate amounts are not provided in a totally vegetarian diet. Ask your doctor about this supplement. You will need to combine your protein foods carefully so that they complement each other, to ensure a high quality protein diet. Three good combinations are:

1 Cereal foods (rice, corn, bread, pasta, barley, oats, wheat, breakfast cereal) with legumes (dried peas, dried beans, lentils) and nuts.
2 Cereal foods with milk or milk products.
3 Seeds (sesame or sunflower seeds) with legumes or nuts.

If you do not drink milk or eat cheese or yoghurt you may need a calcium supplement. Iron supplements are recommended for all vegetarians as the vegetarian diet does not include red meat, a major source of iron.

TAKE-AWAY AND CONVENIENCE FOODS

These foods can provide variety in the diet, but you should avoid foods which are high in fat and be sure to include vegetables and salad with the meal. Chinese meals, chicken with coleslaw, hamburgers with lettuce and tomato, steak sandwiches, jaffles, fish and chips (in moderation) with salad all fall into this category.

EDUCATION *for* PARENTHOOD

Community classes, hospital classes and books as well as nursing staff, doctors and physiotherapists are all possible sources of information.

Most women and their partners rely on a selection from these alternatives. Usually they are encouraged to take part in such programmes, as participation in them broadens the understanding of the physiological processes of pregnancy and labour. As a rule, understanding diminishes anxiety, which is without a doubt the greatest single contributor to a difficult pregnancy and labour.

Most hospitals with obstetrical beds hold parent education classes which can be attended by the woman and her partner. These are also provided in community health centres, early childhood centres and many physiotherapy practices.

Very popular classes are organised by consumer groups such as the Childbirth Education Association of Australia and Parents Centres of Australia.

Vegetarians must plan their diet carefully
▼▼▼

Knowledge is not dangerous
▼▼▼

LABOUR PREPARATION CLASSES

Classes on preparing for labour were begun in 1938 by shrewd physicians and physiotherapists. Although the format has altered somewhat since then, the basic purpose still remains to impart knowledge, teach skills and instil confidence in order to assist women in giving birth.

It helps to meet other people
▼▼▼

BENEFITS OF GROUP ACTIVITY

The fact that preparation for labour is taught in classes rather than by individual instruction is important (although individual attention may of course be given with a class). Pregnancy is an emotional 'high' in a woman's life so she can be more introspective than usual and her emotional and physical needs are greater. Meeting a group of other women who are experiencing the same feelings, fears and frustrations can be a tremendous support. As well as talking with the class leader, it also helps to talk to the other members of the group.

Hospital-based classes have the advantage of having prospective parents associate the hospital with thoughts of well-being rather than illness.

Exercise before the birth will help you regain shape afterwards
▼▼▼

WHEN TO START EXERCISING

The question of exercise is one that commonly arises quite early in pregnancy, especially after the tiredness of the first three months has abated. There are two very simple rules to follow: do nothing that hurts, and do not overdo anything. By following these simple guidelines the risk of doing the wrong thing is practically eliminated.

BREAST EXERCISES

From the fourth month onward the breasts become fuller. As the weight of the breasts increases, they and their muscular supports will have strains placed on them and so it is advisable to support the breasts adequately during pregnancy. However, it is equally important to maintain the tone of the breast muscles to prevent sagging and this can be done by practising two easy but most effective exercises.

1   Bend your elbows, put the palms of your hands together and press them against each other.

2   Fold your arms and press the palms of your hands against your upper arms.

ABDOMINAL EXERCISES

The abdominal muscles have a tremendous ability to stretch. Many a woman looks at her abdomen after her baby is born and wonders about this. Despite this ability, care should be taken to maintain good tone in these muscles so that good body function and good shape can be regained after the baby's birth. No new muscles are provided for pregnancy, nor are there any replacements afterwards.

The function of the abdominal muscles is to support the abdominal organs and perform movement. During the second stage of labour they have great importance in pushing (see Chapter 10: *Is it alright if I push?*).

The abdominal musculature is very similar to a girdle with the fibres running in different directions. Superficially the two long straight muscles from the rib cage to the pelvis run on either side of the navel. Alongside these, two groups of muscles have fibres which run diagonally towards the midline of the body, one group from the rib cage downwards and one from the brim of the pelvis upwards. Lastly and deepest is the muscle layer whose fibres run directly across the abdomen. All these muscles act together to provide support and to initiate movements which will bring the rib cage and pelvic brim closer together, allow rotation of the body, and tightening of the waist.

Exercise need not be complicated to be effective. If you are aware of these muscles, know what they do and how they feel, you can incorporate their movements into all daily activities, exercising them all continuously.

POSTURE

Backache and aching legs are probably two of the most common problems during pregnancy. However, they can be relieved, and in some instances prevented, simply by good posture.

At the beginning of pregnancy, the ligaments supporting the sacro-iliac joints at the back of the pelvis as well as those supporting the lower end of the spine become softer and therefore more lax. As the weight and size of the uterus increases and the woman's abdomen protrudes further, she will automatically increase the curvature of the lower portion of her spine to maintain balance. This is faulty posture and aggravates any tendency to backache. It is correct and common to ascribe this backache to poor posture.

Standing places the greatest strain on muscles and ligaments as pregnancy advances. To counter the weight of the enlarging abdomen, the pelvis should be tilted upwards and backwards, tightening the abdominal muscles and flattening the curve in the lower part of the back. At the same time the head should be held high, the shoulders and arms back and down and the chest a little forward.

Good posture is important not only in standing and walking but also in sitting and lying.

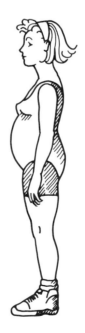

Standing straight helps to prevent backache.

When sitting, the lower part of the back should be supported by the back of a chair or a cushion. Sit upright and take your weight on the backs of your thighs rather than on your buttocks. This position also assists correct breathing and aids digestion.

In late pregnancy, laying on the back for any extended period can lead to a feeling of faintness. This is due to the uterus pressing on the underlying large blood vessels. Lying on your side is the most comfortable position. Also, a higher pillow under the head and shoulders makes breathing easier.

Finally, swollen aching legs are due to sluggish circulation in the legs. Lying with the feet up even for a short time each day is important. A simple method, using an upturned chair and a pillow (see illustration), provides great relief. In this position, bending, stretching and rolling the ankles stimulates the circulation.

Good posture is important ▼▼▼

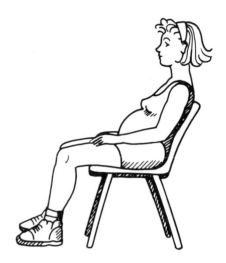

Sitting well aids correct breathing and digestion.

PELVIC FLOOR EXERCISES

The muscles of the pelvic floor are described in some detail in Chapter 9: *How much longer, sister?* Briefly, they lie like a hammock across the opening of the pelvis and support the bladder, the

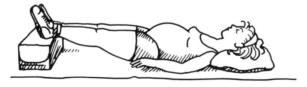

To ease swollen ankles and aching legs, keep your feet up.

uterus and the lower bowel. As the weight of the uterus increases during pregnancy, these muscles come under considerable strain and exercises are needed to maintain their strength and tone. An awareness of these muscles can best be obtained by allowing them to sag down, then consciously tightening them to lift up the pelvic contents. Thinking of the pelvic floor as the floor of a lift being lowered and raised in the body can help. As these muscles tire quickly, exercises should be short but frequent. They can be done in any position, lying, sitting or standing.

CONTROLLED BREATHING

The enlarging uterus tends to interfere with the movements of the diaphragm in breathing, and tightening the abdominal muscles increases this interference by pushing the uterus even higher.

Pregnant women need to learn costal breathing. This method uses the muscles between the ribs to open and close the chest, at the same time relaxing the abdominal muscles in order to allow as much movement as possible in the diaphragm.

During the first stage of labour, before the cervix has opened completely, this breathing ensures an adequate supply of oxygen to the mother and baby. This 'controlled' breathing — breathe in, breathe out, and let go — releases all muscular tensions in the abdomen and is the basic pattern used during first stage contractions.

As the contractions increase in length and intensity they become more painful, making it much more difficult to control the breathing. At this stage, breathing patterns need to be adjusted to allow the mother to cope. Breathing becomes shallower as the contractions intensify but still an 'in, out and let go' routine is used. This requires a lot of skill, concentration, practice and also a knowledge of the stages of labour.

Prenatal classes provide a rehearsal for labour where those skills can be learned and practised.

RELAXATION

The ability to relax and to ease both muscular and emotional tensions comes naturally to some people. Others must learn, and prenatal classes provide an ideal situation to identify the tension areas in the body and to develop the skill of total body relaxation.

Once learned and successfully used during labour, this skill remains a useful mechanism for coping with the many stresses and strains of life.

Controlled breathing is helpful during labour
▼▼▼

CHAPTER 6

EVERYBODY TELLS ME SOMETHING DIFFERENT

The Course of Normal Pregnancy

The one thing that is certain about pregnancy is that the course of each one will be different and that each woman will react in a different way. It is because of these differences that confusion arises.

Many women who have had two, three or more babies naturally regard themselves as authorities on childbirth and their advice to women having their first babies is highly coloured by their own experiences. It is from this pool of anecdotal

What to believe
▼▼▼

information that most confusion emerges. This information often carries messages of doom and despair and is extremely destructive to the confidence of pregnant women.

In many tales there may once have been a tiny grain of truth, but the years of telling and embellishing have buried it in the mumbo-jumbo of superstition.

It is hoped that the facts contained in this chapter will allow you and your partner to decide for yourselves what 'advice' is relevant to you. If nothing else, it should provide the background knowledge for you to talk with your doctor when doubt exists. A statement made by many young mothers after the first pregnancy is that they did not know what questions to ask. Often during the second pregnancy they do not need to ask the questions because they have found out the answers the hard way.

The growth and development of a baby within the uterus produces many changes in the mother's pelvic organs, breasts, lungs, heart and circulation, as well as in total body function. While the female body is designed to cope with pregnancy and the whole process is simply a variation of normal functioning, a knowledge and understanding of the changes can nevertheless greatly reduce the normal anxiety that accompanies pregnancy.

BODY *of the* WOMB (UTERUS)

The uterine body is composed of a mixture of muscle and a little fibrous tissue. The muscle fibres are arranged in layers which pass around the uterus in different directions. The walls of the uterus are 2 to 3 cm thick. There is no voluntary control over the muscle of the uterus, unlike the muscles of our arms and legs over which we have conscious control. The muscle of the uterus is therefore similar to the involuntary muscle of the intestine, blood vessels and the very specialised muscle of the heart.

That is to say, it has an inherent capacity to tighten and relax in a regular fashion.

During pregnancy the uterus enlarges from the size of a small clenched fist to an organ which stretches from within the pelvis up to the ribs. Its weight increases 20 times, from approximately 40 g to 800 g. There is only a slight increase in the number of muscle cells in the uterus during pregnancy; the increase in the weight and size of the uterus is due to an increase in the size of the existing muscle cells.

It is difficult to diagnose a pregnancy by clinical examination before six weeks have passed from the first day of the last menstrual period. At six weeks the uterus begins to feel soft and larger, although it may not be possible to detect these changes in an overweight woman until several weeks later. The uterus grows at a predictable rate throughout pregnancy and the regular checks which are made on its size help to confirm that the pregnancy is progressing and that the baby is growing normally. Any change in the expected rate of growth may be the first sign of a deviation from the normal course of pregnancy, making the doctor aware of the possibility of a multiple pregnancy on the one hand or a slowing in the growth of the baby on the other.

The uterus is the size of a lemon at six to eight weeks, an orange at eight to 10 weeks and a grapefruit by 12 to14 weeks, by which time it can be felt for the first time above the bones at the front of the pelvis. It then grows steadily to reach the umbilicus (navel) by 20 to 24 weeks.

The uterus has a rhythm of its own
▼▼▼

The pregnant uterus should grow at a steady rate
▼▼▼

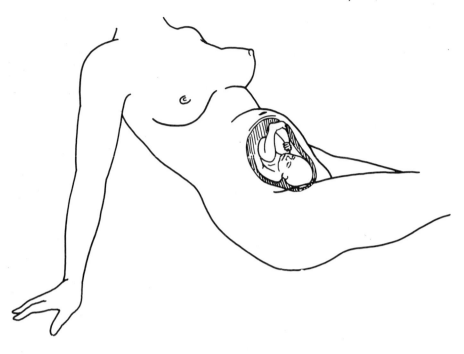

The uterus grows upwards and outwards

▼▼▼

By 30 to 32 weeks it is lying halfway between the umbilicus and the lower margin of the ribs and reaches the lower margin of the ribs at 34 to 36 weeks. These stages are not absolute, and they depend on the amount of fluid within the uterus, the size of the baby, and whether the baby is lying along the lengthways axis (the normal position) of the uterus or transversely across the abdomen.

The uterus not only grows up out of the pelvis towards the ribs but of course also grows outwards. The anterior abdominal wall becomes progressively more stretched as the pregnancy progresses so that in many women by 34 weeks, the umbilicus is no longer a dimple but has become flattened or even everted and remains so during the rest of the pregnancy, returning to normal after delivery.

A woman having her first baby often experiences a feeling termed 'lightening' at about 36 weeks when the leading part of the baby (usually the head) descends into the cavity of the pelvis. When the greatest diameter of the head has passed the brim of the pelvis, it is said to be 'engaged'. The engagement of the head is accompanied by a lowering of the upper border of the uterus, thus reducing the sensation of fullness or pressure under the lower ribs.

The other result of 'lightening', however, is that the baby's head fills the pelvis and applies more pressure on the bladder and the lower part of the bowel, producing a desire to empty the bladder more frequently.

unless there has been damage to one of the blood vessels carrying blood from the baby, an event which is extremely rare. However, when the placenta separates from the uterus after the delivery of the baby there will usually be some fetal blood cells released into the mother's circulation. It is these red cells which may lead to Rhesus sensitisation in women with the Rhesus negative blood group (see Chapter 7: *Is there something wrong, doctor?*).

The umbilical cord contains three blood vessels. Two are arteries carrying blood from the baby to the placenta to discharge the baby's waste products. Unlike arteries in adults, these arteries carry oxygen-depleted blood. The other vessel in the cord is a vein carrying oxygen and nutrient-rich blood back to the baby. This circulation is well established by 10 weeks.

The embryo usually attaches itself to the wall of the uterus near the top. Occasionally, however, it attaches to the lower part of the uterus and the placenta may then form close to or even over the cervix. This condition is called placenta praevia and is one of the causes of bleeding during pregnancy (see Chapter 7: *Is there something wrong, doctor?*).

The placenta grows steadily throughout the pregnancy. During the fourth month it is 7 to 8 cm in diameter, whereas at the end of pregnancy it is 18 to 20 cm in diameter, is 3 cm thick, and weighs 500 to 900 g. It grows in proportion to the baby, being approximately one-sixth of its weight. The bigger the baby, the more nutrients are required to be passed across the placenta.

Complications of pregnancy can cause early dysfunction of the placenta, making it unable to maintain its supply of nutrients and oxygen to the growing baby. If the complication is severe, the supply of nutrients and oxygen may decrease, resulting in either a decreased rate of growth or actual cessation of growth in the developing baby.

Most of the substances carried in the mother's blood, including drugs, are able to pass across the placenta to the baby.

MEMBRANES

These consist of two very thin structures called the amnion and the chorion, which line the uterine cavity. They contain fluid called amniotic fluid (liquor amnii) which surrounds the baby. It is these membranes which rupture during labour and result in the release of fluid commonly referred to as 'breaking of

The position of the placenta ▼▼▼

A healthy placenta means a healthy baby ▼▼▼

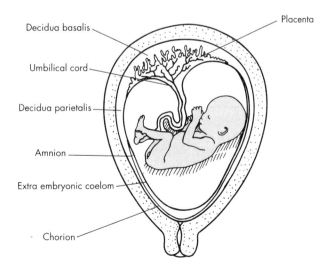

Fetal membranes at 12 weeks

Decidua basalis

Umbilical cord

Decidua parietalis

Amnion

Extra embryonic coelom

Chorion

Placenta

the waters'. The membranes are attached to the placenta and are delivered together with the placenta after the birth of the baby.

AMNIOTIC FLUID

This watery fluid fills the sac of membranes. At term there is approximately 500 to 1000 ml of fluid. It helps maintain a constant temperature within the uterus and gives the developing baby room to move freely until 30 to 34 weeks (after this time the baby is relatively larger and tends to remain in the same general position until delivery).

The fluid also acts as a buffer against any external blow, so that it is almost impossible for the developing baby to be injured by direct force.

The amniotic fluid is produced by the passage of water, salts and other constituents across the placenta and membranes so there is a constant change in the fluid around the baby. Fluid from the baby's lungs and its urine also add to the volume of fluid.

The baby swallows the liquor and this is thought to aid the development of the mouth and muscles of the throat. The amniotic fluid also provides the means of excretion of some of the waste products, although most of these are passed by the umbilical arteries to the placenta to be excreted by the mother. It is this fluid which is tested by amniocentesis to detect some of the abnormalities which occur in pregnancy.

BREASTS

Growth in size of the breasts produces sensations of fullness and activity, some of the earliest symptoms of pregnancy. These may be felt as tingling or tenderness of the breasts or an increased sensitivity of the nipples. Early in pregnancy there is an increase in the blood supply which commonly results in the appearance of blue streaks, as veins become visible through the skin of the breasts. The greater blood flow is necessary to supply the increased amount of glandular tissue and the increased activity in the glands. This activity also extends into the breast tissue which is present in the armpits and may produce obvious swellings. Many women do not realise this is breast tissue and may become unnecessarily concerned about an innocent swelling in this area.

As already described in Chapter 4: *And this* ..., the areola becomes darker, and small lumps often develop around the enlarging nipple, especially in first pregnancies.

As the breasts become heavier they require more support to be comfortable and to prevent the stretching of the fibrous tissue which is responsible for the normal shape of the breasts.

The milky secretion colostrum may become obvious as droplets on the nipple, especially when the breast is stimulated, from approximately 20 weeks. However, some women cannot produce any secretion from the nipple until after the baby is born.

This does not mean they will not be able to breastfeed. The usual reason for this lack of secretion is an inefficient method of expressing the colostrum.

BLOOD *and* CIRCULATION

Major changes occur in the blood and circulation during pregnancy; they are important for the continued growth of the baby.

PLASMA

Plasma, the non-cellular or fluid component of blood, will have increased in volume by an extra one-third at 21 to 24 weeks, and by about an extra half by the end of pregnancy. Before pregnancy the average plasma volume is 2750 ml and an additional 1250 ml is produced in pregnancy. There is a greater increase in women who have had previous pregnancies, and in multiple pregnancies.

Marked decreases occur soon after delivery, through the excretion of urine. This rapidly reduces the plasma volume so that by the fourth week after delivery the volume of the plasma has returned to a normal level.

RED BLOOD CELL VOLUME

This is the volume that would be occupied by the red blood cells if they were separated from the plasma. Red blood cells are the cells which carry oxygen from the lungs to the tissues and, during pregnancy, to the placenta where it is transferred to the baby's red cells. The red blood cell volume increases by approximately 400 ml (from 1400 ml to about 1800 ml) in a single pregnancy, by as much as 700 ml in a twin pregnancy, and by almost a litre in a triplet pregnancy.

CIRCULATION

The work of the heart is also increased in pregnancy. The amount of blood pumped by the heart increases rapidly up to 12 weeks, then gradually up to 32 to 34 weeks, and then remains much the same until term. The total increase is approximately 45 per cent above the pre-pregnancy level. The increased blood flow is mainly due to more blood being pushed forward by each beat of the heart but there is also a gradual increase in the number of heart-beats per minute (pulse rate), so that by term the heart is beating an extra 15 times each minute. Many pregnant women may become aware of their heartbeats for the first time during pregnancy; they describe the sensation as throbbing in the head or chest, as the force of each beat is stronger. Some women also notice short episodes of very rapid beats (palpitations) as during pregnancy the heart is more sensitive to stimuli which increase its rate of beating even more. These are only short episodes and usually require no treatment, returning to normal very quickly.

Blood volume increases during pregnancy
▼▼▼

The heart beats faster during pregnancy
▼▼▼

There is an increase in the number and diameter of the blood vessels in the breast and pelvis, especially those supplying the uterus and particularly those passing into the area where the placenta is attached.

The rapid and prolonged rise in the hormones oestrogen and progesterone in pregnancy result in a relaxation of the muscle cells in the walls of the veins which then become more dilated. Any pre-existing dilated or varicose veins become more prominent. The high levels of oestrogen also produce spider naevi in the skin of some women. These are small red spots on the skin and if inspected closely they will be seen to consist of fine vessels radiating from a central spot or larger vessel in much the same way as a spider is surrounded by its legs; hence the name spider naevi. It is impossible to prevent their appearance although not every woman develops them during pregnancy. They are harmless and fade after birth.

As the pregnant uterus enlarges and becomes heavier, its weight compresses the large veins on the back wall of the abdomen which carry the blood from the lower half of the body back to the heart. When a pregnant woman lies on her back, the compression may reduce the blood flow to such a degree that she feels faint unless she rolls over on her side. This relieves the pressure on the veins and allows the blood flow to return to normal.

Blood pressure may decrease in early pregnancy, but it is usually only by a small amount and is perfectly normal. However, it may lead to a feeling of faintness if blood is allowed to pool in the leg veins when standing still for some time or after rising quickly from a sitting or lying position. As the amount of blood circulating increases, with moving the legs and contracting the leg muscles, the blood pressure returns to normal — if not, the woman should lie down again.

LUNGS

The workload of the lungs changes less than that of the heart during pregnancy. However, the respiratory rate (the number of breaths taken per minute) increases slightly throughout pregnancy.

Towards the end of pregnancy the movement of the diaphragm is restricted by the enlarging uterus. The ribs tend to splay out and the muscles which control the ribs become more important than the diaphragm in moving the air in and out of the lungs. Bad posture makes the muscles less efficient and may make breathing an effort. If the back is kept straight and the shoulders relaxed, the rib muscles can act more efficiently, and the rib cage is often more comfortable.

SKELETON *and* LIGAMENTS

Many changes occur in pregnancy. The hormones which cause relaxation of the muscles in the veins also soften the ligaments which support the joints of the pelvis, allowing the ligaments to stretch. This has the advantage of making the pelvis supple and possibly allowing it to become slightly larger to allow the baby through. However, the disadvantage is that it is easy to strain these joints. This is especially common in the sacro-iliac joints at the back of the pelvis which may be strained by lifting heavy objects or by lifting incorrectly. The joint at the front of the pelvis, called the symphysis pubis, may also be involved and the separation here may be recognised as a widening of the gap where the two pelvic bones meet. If either of these areas widen more than usual they may produce pain. A typical example of ligament-softening is sciatica, when the lower vertebrae of the spine and sacro-iliac joints are involved. Any woman who had back problems before pregnancy will have to pay particular attention to her posture to avoid aggravating any weakness while the ligaments which support these joints are relaxed.

The enlarging uterus tends to alter the centre of gravity of the body. To compensate for this there is a tendency to accentuate the natural hollow in the lower back. This tilts the pelvis backwards and places extra strain on the back, the hips and the back of the legs. To compensate for the unnatural posture, each step becomes shorter, producing the characteristic 'pregnancy waddle'. This can be prevented by correct posture (see Chapter 5: *Is everything all right?*).

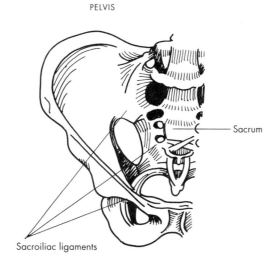

PELVIS

Sacrum

Sacroiliac ligaments

METABOLISM

Weight gain in pregnancy varies from woman to woman and from pregnancy to pregnancy and depends partly upon the original body build. Weight gain in pregnancy is distributed thus:

	KG
Baby	3.0-3.5
Placenta	0.6-0.7
Amniotic fluid	0.6-1.0
Increase in weight of uterus	0.8
Increase in weight of breasts	0.5-0.7
Increase in weight of blood	1.5-2.0
Total (excluding fat and fluid retention)	7.0-8.7

There is also an increase in fluid retention and in fat deposition. The excess fluid is lost soon after delivery and fat deposition is used up during breastfeeding. However, if more than 10 kg are gained during pregnancy the mother will be heavier after the baby is born than she was before the pregnancy. Most of the extra weight will be in the form of extra fatty tissue, storage for use at a later time.

MULTIPLE PREGNANCY

A multiple pregnancy accentuates all the changes of pregnancy, and these changes occur more dramatically at an earlier stage than in a single pregnancy. In particular, the pressure symptoms of the enlarging uterus are more marked with a multiple pregnancy. For example, at 32 to 34 weeks many mothers with twins have a uterus as big, if not bigger, than the average term size of a single pregnancy. Body weight is increased correspondingly and the requirements for iron and all the other nutrients necessary for the development of the fetuses are also increased.

GROWTH *and* DEVELOPMENT *of the* FETUS

In the past methods of detecting fetal growth relied on abdominal examination and measurement. Estimates of the age of the fetus calculated from the first day of the last menstrual period can be quite inaccurate, particularly if the menstrual cycles are irregular. Pregnancies occurring soon after stopping taking oral contraceptives are also difficult to date accurately.

In the last 20 years the use of ultrasound in pregnancy has expanded the knowledge of fetal growth and has provided a safe technique for establishing the age of the fetus.

When doubt exists about the duration of pregnancy, this simple, non-invasive test in the first half of the pregnancy can clarify the problem with a high degree of accuracy.

In the first three months of pregnancy ultrasound can be used to measure the length of the embryo and accurately date its age. In the second three months it can also be used to measure reliably the size of the fetal head and trunk and provide accurate dates up to 20 weeks and in most cases the parents can be reassured that their baby is developing normally.

In the last three months, regular measurements of the head and trunk can confirm the normal rate of growth of the fetus and identify those cases where the growth rate is abnormal. For example, women with diabetes may have fetuses that grow too rapidly. Women with blood pressure problems on the other hand may have placental dysfunction that will lead to slowed growth of the baby.

Note that frequently the size of the baby in late pregnancy is reported as being 'x' weeks size. This does not mean that the pregnancy is 'x' weeks, but rather that the baby is the size usually seen at 'x' weeks of pregnancy.

In cases of bleeding in pregnancy, the use of ultrasound enables the position of the placenta to be accurately located. Placenta praevia can thus be diagnosed and correct decisions about treatment can therefore be made in advance.

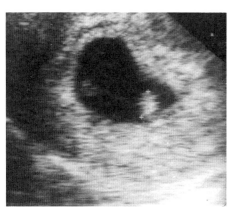

Sac containing embryo and yolk sac seen on vaginal ultrasound.

HOW ULTRASOUND WORKS

Ultrasound, which is sound beyond the range of human hearing, can be used very effectively for demonstrating structures within the human body. Just as a hammer hitting a gong produces sound, so an electrical voltage applied to a special ceramic crystal called a transducer produces ultrasound. Little ultrasonic waves lasting one three-millionth part of a second are repeated 500 times a second. These are sent as a beam to search the body cavities in a process which is rather like exploring a darkened room with the light beam from a torch. Some of the sound is reflected as echoes from boundaries between structures such as the uterus and placenta or from the internal structures within the baby. The echoes are received by the transducer and are displayed as tens of thousands of tiny spots of light which together build a two-dimensional picture on the screen of a television monitor. From this, photographs are made for future reference. A three-dimensional picture of the baby and its environment is obtained by moving the transducer along different planes of section to look at the baby from several angles. Ultrasound is safe at the energy levels used in medical practice, and considerable scrutiny over many years by numerous investigators has revealed no human injury attributable to it. In fact, at much greater energy levels no harmful effects have been found and there is no ionising radiation involved.

FETAL GROWTH

It has been shown in Chapter 2: *How does our baby grow?* that embryonic development is virtually complete by eight weeks after fertilisation (10 weeks of amenorrhoea).

During the first week the germinal cells divide. In the second week the ectoderm and endoderm differentiate and in the third week the mesoderm appears. While this is happening, there is enormous growth of the placental tissue to provide the growing embryo with food and oxygen, and the amniotic sac grows rapidly to encase the delicate embryo in a protective fluid-filled envelope. Indeed from this stage the placental growth far outstrips the embryonic growth (until by 12 weeks the placenta is six times the weight of the fetus).

At four weeks the somites start to develop and the heart begins to beat. Between four and eight weeks there is rapid differentiation of the embryo into an essentially human appearance. The embryo is motionless in the first seven weeks of life, and it grows about 1 mm a day up to the end of eight weeks. At eight weeks the embryo weighs a mere 1 g and is 2.5 cm long.

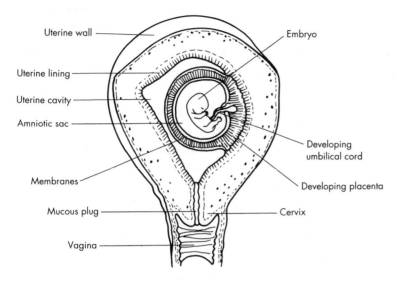

Uterine wall
Uterine lining
Uterine cavity
Amniotic sac
Membranes
Mucous plug
Vagina
Embryo
Developing umbilical cord
Developing placenta
Cervix

Eight weeks (about 2.5 cm long)

Twelve weeks (about 5 cm long)

Fetal development ▼▼▼

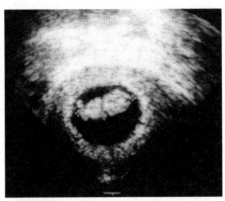

Ultrasound showing early embryo at around 8 weeks pregnancy.

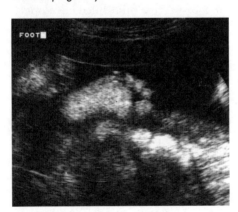

Ultrasound showing foot, 12 weeks.

By 12 weeks the fetus weighs 14 g and is 7 cm long, but its sex cannot yet be determined by external examination. Between eight and 12 weeks the circulation attains its full fetal development. Subsequent fetal growth is then usually measured as total length, from the top of the head to the heels, and is known as 'crown-heel length' or 'standing height'. The average 'height' at birth is 50 cm (approximately 20 in) and average weight is 3250 g (approximately 7 lb 3 oz). The growth in length is steady, whereas the weight does not increase as rapidly until after 30 weeks. Indeed in the last eight weeks, the weight of the fetus doubles but its length increases by only one-fifth.

No attempt will be made here to describe the changes that occur week by week in the last 30 weeks. Instead a description will be given of the stage of growth reached at 14 weeks, 18 weeks, 24 weeks, 34 weeks and 40 weeks.

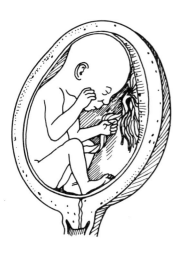

Twenty weeks (25 cm long)

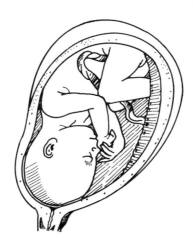

Twenty-four weeks (about 32 cm long)

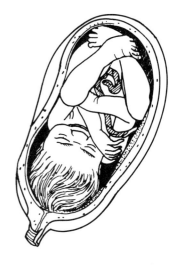

Thirty-six weeks (44–45 cm long)

Fourteen weeks

The fetus floats in a sac of liquor amnii several times greater than its own size, and is attached to the placenta by a long umbilical cord. The fetus is 8.5 cm long and weighs 50 g. The head has grown more than the body and looks disproportionately large. The legs and arms are thin and spindly but the thighs and toes are well formed and the nails are present. It is usually possible to tell the sex from the external genital organs.

Swallowing movements appear at about 12 to 14 weeks and from then on the fetus swallows liquor and secretes small quantities of urine. Soon after this the enzymes and ferments of the digestive tract begin to appear, as the stomach and intestines are now completely formed.

Bile is formed at about 12 weeks, and by 16 weeks meconium, a dark green viscid substance composed of bile, intestinal juices and swallowed skin cells, is present in the fetal

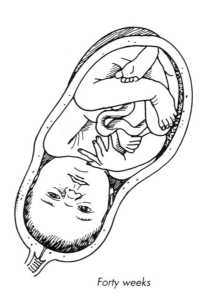

Forty weeks

intestine. Although breathing motions can be seen as early as 14 weeks, the lungs will not have developed sufficiently to allow life outside the uterus until 27 to 28 weeks. All the endocrine glands (the pituitary, the thyroid, the gonads and the adrenals) are formed and all except the gonads have commenced functioning.

The skeletal and muscular systems are well developed and the

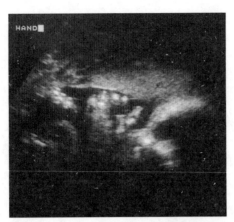
Ultrasound showing hand, 16 weeks.

*Fetal
movements
vary in
different
women*
▼▼▼

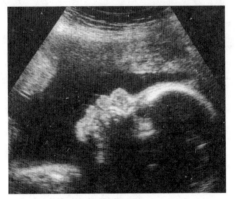
Ultrasound showing facial profile, 16 weeks.

about 30 cm long and weighs less than 230 g. Its face is broad and flat and the eyes widely separated. The eyelids are present but fused together. The ear can be recognised as a dimple, surrounded by an elliptical ridge which will form the external ear. The skin everywhere is bright pink and transparent and covered with fine down-like hair, called lanugo. There are a few true hairs on the front of the head. The heart is beating strongly, but is usually not able to be heard through the mother's abdominal wall for another month.

Fetal movement or 'quickening' is usually noticed at about 18 to 20 weeks. It is sometimes later with the first baby, sometimes a little earlier with the second and third. Detecting the movement depends to some extent on the thickness of the abdominal wall and the position of the placenta. If the placenta is on the anterior uterine wall, it may mask the baby's movements for two or three weeks.

Once they have started, fetal movements greatly increase in frequency and intensity over the next few weeks. Soon after 20 weeks there is often a decrease in fetal activity which may be a source of anxiety to individual women. Remember, however, that fetal movements are very varied and that not all movements can be felt strongly by all pregnant women. There is evidence that excitement and stress in pregnant women can produce greater activity in the baby, possibly through the liberation of adrenaline and other hormones.

brain has established nervous connections with quite a few of the muscles of the arms and legs. Isolated muscle movements have been occurring from as early as 10 weeks, and by 12 weeks arm and leg movements similar to swimming can be produced by stimulating the back of the fetus. However, these are not usually recognised by the pregnant woman until 18 weeks when they are felt as faint tapping sensations in the lower abdomen.

Eighteen weeks
The fetus is floating freely in about 300 ml of liquor amnii. The placenta at this stage is relatively large, weighing 120 to 140 g. The fetus is

Twenty-four weeks

At 24 weeks the fetus has increased in length to between 27 and 35 cm and weighs about 700 g. The placenta weighs about 240 g and the fetus is surrounded by some 500 ml of liquor amnii.

The parts of the body, the head, back buttocks and limbs, can be distinguished by touch and the heart sounds can be clearly heard with a stethoscope, or by placing one ear to the abdomen, over the fetal back.

The skin of the fetus is wrinkled and red and is covered with a heavy coating of a white creamy material derived from the activity of the sebaceous glands of the skin. This layer, known as the vernix caseosa, persists until birth, and prevents the skin becoming waterlogged by the constant exposure to the amniotic fluid. The wrinkling of the skin is apparently due to the rapid rate of skin growth at this stage and to the lack of fat beneath the skin.

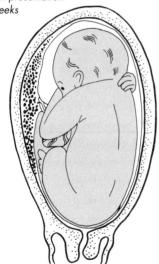

Breech presentation
28 weeks

The eyelids are separated and the eyelashes and eyebrows are forming. The face is much more infant-like and the hair over the trunk is darker. By this time a relatively large increase in growth of the fetus's lower abdominal wall has occurred, bringing the attachment of the umbilical cord at the navel, more nearly into the middle of its abdomen. Between 18 and 20 weeks, active breathing movements occur and the amniotic fluid tides in and out of the fetal lungs. This may indeed assist lung growth and development. From 28 weeks on, these breathing movements decrease, possibly because the liquor begins to contain too much debris, such as lanugo hairs and skin cells shed from the baby, which might block the air passages after it is born. By 28 weeks active sucking can and does occur inside the uterus and the fetus has often been shown by ultrasound to be sucking its thumb or fingers.

At 28 weeks the fetus has a good chance of survival, should labour occur then, and traditionally this has been regarded as the stage of viability. The survival of such a pre-term baby weighing approximately 1 kg depends on a variety of factors such as the length of labour, the method of delivery and placental function at the time. It is far preferable for women in pre-term labour to be transferred to units where specialised facilities exist, prior to the birth of the baby.

Under such conditions, the survival rate at 28 weeks can be as high as 85 per cent and up to 65 per cent at 26 weeks. For most practical

Intensive care for a pre-term baby
▼▼▼

purposes it now appears that the 26 week fetus weighing 700 g (approximately 1½ lb) represents the lower limit of survival, but there are exceptions. Sometimes infants apparently less mature than 26 weeks survive, but many of these would be smaller than average infants, who are actually more mature than their weight or length would indicate; the reverse, of course, is also true.

Between 28 and 37 weeks the amount of liquor amnii increases to about 1 to 1½ litres. Thereafter it slowly decreases, leaving less room for the fetus to move about. Its movements become larger and it is able to turn around completely from a breech to a head presentation. This turning, known as version, usually finishes by 34 weeks, but occasionally occurs up to the onset of labour.

Thirty-four weeks

The fetus at 34 weeks, six weeks before full term, is quite long, measuring 42 cm but still weighs only 2 kg. In the next six weeks it will almost double its weight while gaining an extra 5 to 7 cm in length. The bones of the head are soft and pliable. The skin is still bright pink, but most of the lanugo has been shed from the body. Although still thin and wrinkled it has some subcutaneous fat.

It has a very good chance of survival if born now, but would need specialised care for up to one month. The biggest problem in all pre-term babies is heat regulation. Such an infant needs to spend the first few weeks of its life in the warm moist air of a humidicrib.

In the last six weeks of pregnancy the amount of fetal movement depends mainly on the amount of liquor amnii present and the laxity of the mother's abdominal muscles.

Forty weeks

At term, the fetus is said to have reached maturity. The average weight is 3250 g (7 lb 3 oz), boys being slightly heavier than girls, and the average length is 50 cm (20 in). This is also the average length of the umbilical cord, although great variations occur in length, thickness and tortuosity of the cord.

The placenta at term measures 18 to 20 cm in diameter, is 3 cm thick at its centre, and weighs between 450 and 700 g.

The weight of the fetus at term may vary between about 2700 g (6 lb) and about 4500 g (10 lb) depending on the genetic characteristics inherited from its parents and the degree of nutrition supplied by the placenta. The amount of weight that the mother gains during the pregnancy has little effect on the weight of the baby, although it is true that maternal malnutrition can produce a thin baby. It has now been

Pre-term babies need to be kept warm
▼▼▼

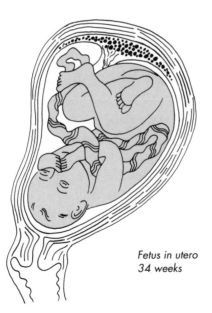

Fetus in utero
34 weeks

definitely shown that smoking during pregnancy has the same effect, possibly by reducing the blood flow through the uterus and placenta.

Inside the uterus, the fetus is usually still covered by a thick white creamy coat of vernix caseosa, and the amount of liquor amnii has decreased to between 570 and 1130 ml. The skin is smooth and pink and the fetus is plump with abundant subcutaneous fat, often in rolls at the neck line and the lower abdomen. The body hair has disappeared except over the shoulders. The hair on the head may be thin and scanty or thick and abundant. The bones of the head are thicker and close together, although they are not fused; the soft spot in front (anterior fontanelle) is not covered by bone.

The attitude of the fetus is described as one of uniform flexion: the head is bent forwards with the chin on the chest; the arms are bent and folded across the chest and the hips and knees are bent; and the feet lie, in many cases crossed, in front of the lower abdomen and genital organs. In this position, the fetus forms an egg-shaped oval, the smaller end being the head, which usually lies within the mother's pelvis. In about 3 per cent of pregnancies, the baby's buttocks lie in or over the pelvic cavity; this is known as a breech presentation (see Chapter 5: *Is there something wrong, doctor?*).

CHAPTER 7

IS THERE SOMETHING WRONG, DOCTOR?

Problem Pregnancies

'Problem pregnancies' is the term used to describe pregnancies in which there is a greater than usual chance of problems arising from either the woman, her baby, or both.

Exhaustive lists can be made up of such situations by including slight variations from normal, but this chapter will deal with a few of the most common situations which are well known to lead to an unsuccessful pregnancy if they go undetected and are therefore not dealt with correctly.

Problems may occur in about 10 per cent of pregnancies

▼▼▼

Broadly speaking, problems which can place a pregnancy at risk can be divided into two groups:

1 Conditions occurring for the first time during a pregnancy which are directly attributable to that pregnancy, and

2 Conditions occurring before the pregnancy began which may become more severe as the pregnancy progresses.

There is a small overlap between these two groups and there are some situations which cannot be placed in either of these categories.

Conditions Attributable *to* Pregnancy

Hypertension associated with pregnancy

Hypertension, or pre-eclampsia, is more popularly but incorrectly named pre-eclamptic toxaemia. Its signs are high blood pressure, swelling of the hands and feet and presence of protein in the urine.

The precise cause is not known. It is most common in first pregnancies and multiple pregnancies. It does not usually recur in subsequent pregnancies and is more common if the mother is under 18 years or over 35 years of age. As a rule, it has no symptoms and is only detected by routine recording of blood pressure.

The importance of this condition is that if proper management is not commenced, the level of the blood pressure can rise, in rare cases resulting in the pregnant woman having fits (eclampsia) and, in extreme cases, kidney damage and cerebral haemorrhage. In addition, the blood flow to the uterus slows and the baby does not receive adequate amounts of food and oxygen which will result in it being improperly nourished.

In some cases, bleeding occurs because the placenta separates; this may call for rapid intervention to save the life of mother and baby.

If a rise in blood pressure greater than 140/90 is detected, the best treatment is rest. Usually with bed rest the blood pressure will remain normal, and so allow the pregnancy to continue without harm to mother or baby.

Sometimes the blood pressure will not settle with rest. Often in these cases protein is detected in the woman's urine, which indicates that her kidneys are not functioning adequately.

All these changes will disappear after the birth of the baby.

If the expected date of delivery is near, labour may be induced. If the baby is not due for five weeks or more, drugs to lower the blood pressure can be given without harm to the baby to enable the pregnancy to continue without risk to the mother. In this way a stage may be reached where the baby can be safely delivered and not develop problems associated with immaturity. Until this time, close observations will be kept on the mother and special tests may be performed to confirm that the baby remains in good health (see pages 95–98).

Placental bleeding

Bleeding due to placental separation is called antepartum haemorrhage (APH).

If the placenta is situated in the upper part of the uterus the bleeding is known as accidental (occurring by chance) haemorrhage.

When bleeding is associated with a placenta which is situated in the lower part of the uterus it is called placenta praevia (coming before).

Accidental haemorrhage may be associated with hypertension or it

Bed rest is the best treatment for high blood pressure

▼▼▼

may occur for no apparent reason. Unless the bleeding is severe there is no danger to the mother. However, even small amounts of bleeding and placental separation may cause problems for the baby.

With placenta praevia, uterine contractions cause the placenta to separate slightly. There is usually no pain. Because the bleeding is from the uterus and can be quite heavy it poses more problems for the mother than the baby.

If bleeding occurs your doctor should be notified or if it is obviously heavy, call an ambulance. Admission to hospital is frequently necessary. An ultrasonic examination will help decide whether the placenta is high or low in the uterus.

If a placenta praevia is diagnosed you will probably be advised to remain in hospital as the bleeding will often recur and it may be heavy enough to require a blood transfusion. In such a situation the aim is to observe the mother and her baby until two or three weeks before the expected date of delivery at which time the baby will be delivered by caesarean section.

If the placenta is in the upper part of the uterus, bed rest in hospital is advised until the bleeding has stopped. If there is no recurrence it is usually possible to go home after five or six days. In both instances tests will be performed to determine how the baby is coping with these disturbances (see pages 95–98).

MULTIPLE PREGNANCY

Twins occur in about one in every 90 pregnancies. They are usually suspected when the uterus grows at a faster rate than anticipated. The diagnosis can be confirmed by an ultrasonic examination which will also show the sizes of the babies and the positions in which they are lying at that time.

Pre-term labour is more common in multiple pregnancies and so some obstetricians advise their patients to rest in hospital from 30 to 34 weeks which is a common time for pre-term labour to commence. However there is no evidence that this is effective.

Uniovular twins share a common placenta and one twin may get the majority of the nutrients and oxygen and so be larger. The only way to monitor this accurately is to have ultrasonic examinations performed at

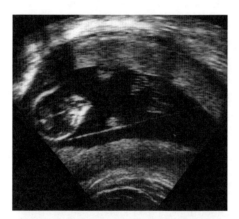

Ultrasound showing twin pregnancy (2 sacs)

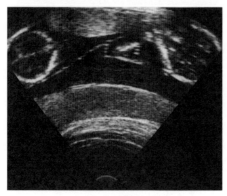

Ultrasound showing early twin pregnancy

intervals to see how the babies are growing. If the growth rate is similar, all is well. If one baby is obviously growing faster than the other, admission to hospital for bed rest and more detailed monitoring of the babies is advisable.

BREECH PRESENTATION

This may be a problem because during delivery the largest part of the baby, the head, comes last. It is also the hardest and least compressible portion of the baby.

Breech labours require more interference on the part of the obstetrician and injury to the baby during delivery is more common, even in the best hands. Some obstetricians try to turn babies to the head-first position before labour commences by manipulating the baby through the mother's abdominal wall, and sometimes they are successful. However, most obstetricians believe that if a baby can turn itself, it will, without any need for manipulation.

It is unusual, although not unheard of, for a baby to turn itself in the last two to three weeks of pregnancy. Once the diagnosis has been suspected it can be confirmed by an ultrasonic examination.

An X-ray examination can measure the size of the woman's pelvis and if it is found to be of above average size a normal labour can be anticipated. Such an examination is not harmful to the baby.

If the pelvis is of average or below average size, a caesarean section may be recommended as the best method of delivery. Caesarean section is a common method of delivering breech babies, especially if they are pre-term or if labour is slow (as this usually implies a large baby).

GROWTH RETARDATION

Babies may be small at birth for any of several reasons:

1   They may be normal but small (this is determined genetically);

2   They may be small because of below-average nourishment;

3   Least commonly, they may be congenitally abnormal;

4   Lastly, they may be born before term (see pages 92 and 103).

Unfortunately, in the first three categories it is impossible in all instances to determine before birth the precise reason for the small size of the baby. If it were possible, there would be no cause for alarm for babies in the first category as they are perfectly normal and have adequate nutrition.

Growth retardation is suspected if the uterus does not grow at a normal rate. Often the woman gains little or no weight and in some instances loses weight. The uterus is smaller because the baby is smaller and because there is less amniotic fluid around the baby than in a normal pregnancy, and the baby is smaller because there is some disorder of the placenta. This situation is important because the baby may die from lack of oxygen before delivery or, more commonly, it may have difficulties during labour which could necessitate delivery by forceps or caesarean section.

The diagnosis of growth retardation can be confirmed by an

'What's that lump under my ribs?'
▼▼▼

'I don't seem very large'
▼▼▼

ultrasonic examination and the rate of growth determined by repeating these examinations at intervals of 14 days.

Again, admission to hospital for bed rest to improve placental blood flow and to check the baby's progress is advised. Delivery is induced when the obstetrician, in the light of clinical information and the investigations, decides that the baby is better off in the nursery than inside its mother. This decision is made in consultation with the parents and a paediatrician.

Surprisingly these babies usually show very few of the problems that one would normally associate with pre-term birth and once feeding is established they rapidly gain weight.

Some pre-term labours can be prevented
▼▼▼

PRE-TERM LABOUR

This is defined as labour commencing before 37 completed weeks. In most instances there is no obvious cause for the labour commencing early, although it may be associated with a twin pregnancy, antepartum haemorrhage or pre-eclampsia.

Sometimes it is due to an uncommon condition called poly-hydramnios where there is an excessive amount of amniotic fluid. Pre-term labour may also be due to congenital malformations of the uterus which prevent it from expanding to its full capacity. Alternatively, it may be associated with an incompetent cervix, that is, one which has lost its ability to hold the pregnancy within the uterus. This situation can arise after a previous normal delivery but, more commonly these days, after a previous abortion

where the cervix was damaged by the necessarily rapid dilatation (especially in terminations after 10 weeks).

Unfortunately the diagnosis of incompetent cervix is not ususally made until the labour is over. However, it can often be prevented from recurring in a future pregnancy by stitching the cervix. This stitch is usually put in place between 10 and 14 weeks and it provides the support that is lacking in the cervix and holds the pregnancy in place. It is usually removed two to three weeks before the expected date of delivery or at the onset of a pre-term labour.

If pre-term labour commences, the woman is admitted to hospital and an assessment is made to see whether or not there is any obvious cause for the labour. If there is no obvious cause, drugs such as Ventolin or Ritodrine can be given intravenously and in a high percentage of cases these temporarily stop the uterus from contracting. The aim is to stop the uterus contracting for one to two days during which time cortisone-type drugs are given to the mother. These drugs cross the placenta and act on the baby's lungs to produce a substance called surfactant. Surfactant is the natural substance which prevents the development of hyaline membrane disease which is the most common cause of sickness and death amongst pre-term babies. It is produced in the baby's air sacs after 35 weeks.

If the pre-term labour is due to antepartum haemorrhage or the mother's high blood pressure, it is unwise to attempt to stop the labour.

CONDITIONS WHICH MAY *be* AGGRAVATED *by* PREGNANCY

HYPERTENSION

A small group of women have high blood pressure before they become pregnant. Of these women, some may never have been pregnant and others may have hypertension as an after-effect of a previous pregnancy. Many of them may be receiving treatment to maintain their blood pressure at normal levels.

The effects of high blood pressure on the mother and baby are similar to the effects of pregnancy-induced hypertension, but treatment usually prevents the blood pressure from rising to such high levels. Drugs used for the treatment of high blood pressure are not thought to cause fetal abnormalities.

Usually the early part of the pregnancy is trouble-free. As the pregnancy progresses, it is common for the blood pressure to fall below the levels recorded at the commencement of the pregnancy. However, it usually rises again around 28 to 30 weeks. Medication is continued and dosages frequently need to be increased. As bed rest is the best treatment, this is often advised towards the end of pregnancy. Bed rest also has the advantage of increasing the blood supply to the uterus and baby. The condition of both the mother and baby is carefully monitored and delivery is usually advised when it is felt that neither the mother nor the baby can benefit further from allowing the pregnancy to continue.

DIABETES

In the early 1950s it was realised that the control of diabetes during pregnancy had to be much stricter than that allowed in patients who were not pregnant. This led to a greatly improved survival rate for babies of diabetic mothers. Today, in the best hands, the mortality rate amongst babies of diabetic mothers is only slightly higher than that of babies whose mothers are not diabetic.

During pregnancy, increasing amounts of insulin are needed to keep the mother's sugar levels within the normal range. This is because some hormones produced by the placenta act against insulin. In order to ensure that the dosage of insulin is correct, it is necessary to check the levels of glucose in the woman's blood frequently and raise or lower the dose of insulin accordingly. The woman, her obstetrician and physician should act in close co-operation. More frequent medical checks are necessary. Admission to hospital may occasionally be necessary to re-establish control of the blood sugar level.

Diabetic patients are able to measure the level of glucose in their own blood using an instrument called a glucometer. This has revolutionised the management of diabetes during pregnancy, reducing the need for diabetic women to be admitted to hospital during the last weeks of pregnancy.

High blood pressure can run in families
▼▼▼

Diabetes must be controlled strictly
▼▼▼

Anti-D
gamma-
globulin has
been a great
advance
▼▼▼

If control of the diabetes is poor, some complications of pregnancy are more likely to occur. These include pregnancy-induced hypertension and hydramnios. In addition, the baby may be unduly large and this could cause problems during labour and delivery. The baby is usually delivered at about 37 or 38 weeks as prolonging the pregnancy beyond this time slightly increases the chances of the baby dying unexpectedly.

There are some women in whom diabetes appears for the first time during pregnancy. This occurs because the placental hormones antagonise the action of the woman's own insulin. Fortunately, this type of pregnancy diabetes can usually be controlled by diet alone. Admission to hospital is not the rule but a close watch needs to be kept on the pregnancy.

Sometimes the diabetes cannot be controlled by diet and the woman will need to be admitted to hospital so that insulin treatment can be commenced. Following this, management of her pregnancy is the same as for a woman who has been on insulin all through her pregnancy. After delivery this pregnancy-induced diabetes disappears. However, about 40 per cent of women with this disorder become diabetic in later years.

OTHER ILLNESSES

As a rule, any woman with a pre-existing illness such as heart or kidney disease or epilepsy will need to have more frequent prenatal visits. Quite often a close check also needs to be maintained by her family doctor as well as by her obstetrician. Usually it is essential that the medication normally taken be continued during pregnancy.

It is felt it is not within the scope of this book to discuss these conditions individually.

RHESUS ISO-IMMUNISATION

This condition occurs in women with Rhesus negative blood who have had previous pregnancies or who have received a blood transfusion in the past. Fortunately, it is a rare occurrence these days due to the introduction of a substance called anti-D gamma-globulin in 1966. When an Rh-negative woman has an Rh-positive baby, some of the baby's blood cells may cross into the mother. Because these cells are foreign to the mother, her body manufactures antibodies against them. In a subsequent pregnancy these antibodies can cross to the baby and if the baby is Rh positive they may attach to its red blood cells and break them down, producing anaemia.

Bleeding from baby to mother can occur at virtually any time during pregnancy. It may occur at the time of an ectopic pregnancy, or a miscarriage, or as a result of abortion or antepartum haemorrhage. However, it most commonly occurs at delivery.

Anti-D gamma-globulin is identical to the antibody produced by the mother and if it is injected into the woman following delivery or miscarriage, it will destroy any Rh-positive blood cells that may have crossed into the woman's circulation.

Occasionally this treatment is not successful and because of this, Rh-negative women should have their blood checked for antibodies at the commencement of each pregnancy and subsequently at around 28 and 36 weeks.

Rh-positive women have the check done in early pregnancy but it is not required later.

If antibodies are detected, it is a sign that the baby may be anaemic and further tests need to be undertaken to determine how severe the anemia is. This is done by examining a sample of amniotic fluid taken by amniocentesis. Depending on the result of the test it may need to be repeated from time to time before the baby is born.

If examination of the amniotic fluid shows that the baby is not anaemic, no changes in the management of the pregnancy are needed. Often, if the baby is thought to be mildly anaemic, labour is induced about two weeks early. In the rare instances where the anaemia is judged to be severe, the baby may need to be delivered six or even eight weeks before the expected date. Sometimes the anaemia is so severe that the baby may need to have a transfusion before it is born.

Immediately following the birth of the baby, a sample of its blood is checked to see whether or not it needs a blood transfusion. In either event it will need to be watched in a special nursery where usually it will be nursed in a crib under a light which helps break down bilirubin. This is a toxic substance produced by the breakdown of blood cells; if allowed to reach high levels it can lead to brain damage.

SPECIAL TESTS USED *in* ASSESSMENT *of the* FETUS

ULTRASOUND

An ultrasonic examination of the uterus is a procedure which is harmless to both mother and baby.

Ultrasound is used in some instances to confirm a diagnosis of pregnancy and it can be useful in determining whether or not the pregnancy has implanted in the uterus or in another site such as a Fallopian tube.

In the first 20 weeks of pregnancy, measurement of the fetus will give a very accurate estimate of how far the pregnancy has progressed. This may be performed for women who have irregular menstrual cycles or those who have conceived immediately after stopping taking a contraceptive pill. It is also helpful in the management of pregnancies in women suffering from Rhesus iso-immunisation, hypertension or diabetes, who may have to deliver early.

If bleeding occurs in early pregnancy and there is some doubt as to whether or not this has harmed the baby, an ultrasonic examination can tell whether or not the baby is the right size and whether or not it is still alive. In late pregnancy it is used to determine whether or not the bleeding is from a placenta situated in the upper part of the uterus or in the lower part of the uterus (placenta praevia) (see pages 89–90).

Some but by no means all fetal abnormalities may be diagnosed by ultrasound in either early or late pregnancy. The abnormality most commonly diagnosed by this method is anencephaly which occurs in about one in 1000 pregnancies.

A diagnosis of twins can be confirmed by an ultrasonic examination, and in situations where there is some doubt as to the baby's position, ultrasound can be most helpful.

In addition, repeated measurements of the baby's size in late pregnancy can show whether or not the baby is growing at a normal rate and provide information as to the position of the placenta and the volume of fluid surrounding the baby.

OESTRIOL AND HUMAN PLACENTAL LACTOGEN (HPL)

The measurement of these two pregnancy hormones has not been useful in the management of problem pregnancies and they are now only rarely used.

CARDIOTOCOGRAPHY

This is the most commonly used test to determine the state of the baby's health. It is a simple test which usually takes from 20 to 30 minutes to perform. The woman lies on a bed and the baby's heart rate is monitored

by ultrasound. A pressure-sensitive disc which determines whether or not the uterus is contracting or if the baby is moving is placed over her uterus.

Babies who are in good health usually move several times during the examination and at the time of movement the baby's heart rate usually increases. This is regarded as normal and means the baby is in no immediate danger. Little or no fetal movement and no variation during the examination may be an indication that the baby is ill. The test will then be repeated in 24 hours.

ANTENATAL DIAGNOSIS

In a small minority of pregnancies, tests to determine whether or not a baby has a specific abnormality may be advised. Most commonly this will occur when a mother is 37 years of age or over and is more likely to have a baby with abnormal chromosomes than a younger woman. The most commonly occurring disorder of chromosomes is Down's Syndrome and about half the children with this problem are born to women over the age of 35. Other disorders which can be diagnosed in the first half of pregnancy include spina bifida, some blood disorders such as thalassaemia, cystic fibrosis and a whole host of rare chemical disorders which are due to genetic deficiencies.

Apart from age the usual reason for having a diagnostic test is because either a couple have had a baby with a specific illness previously or in some instances where there is a family history of hereditary disease which can be diagnosed before birth. Occasionally the parents themselves have abnormal chromosomes which can be passed on to the fetus in a different pattern which could result in great handicap.

There are several methods of antenatal diagnosis available.

Amniocentesis

This involves the withdrawal of fluid from around the baby between 14-16 weeks of the commencement of the last menstrual period. The fluid is obtained by passing a needle through the woman's abdominal wall and the muscle of the uterus into the bag of fluid surrounding the baby. There is a risk of miscarriage following this procedure of between $\frac{1}{2}$ to 1 per cent.

The test will tell whether the baby has normal chromosomes, what its sex is and also it will detect the worst 90 per cent of cases of spina bifida. In addition an ultrasound examination at the same time can detect some other structural abnormalities of the baby. The results of the amniocentesis are available after about three weeks.

Chorionic villous sampling (CVS)

This which involves passing a small tube up through the cervix and removing a small fragment of chorion by gentle suction. Chorion is the tissue from which the placenta develops. This test is done between 10 and 12 weeks after the last period (earlier than amniocentesis) and the result is usually available within 14 days. An ultrasound examination is performed before, during and after the test. Chromosome disorders, some blood disorders and some rare biochemical disorders can be

diagnosed by this technique. This test is not appropriate for people whose primary concern is whether their baby will have spina bifida.

The miscarriage rate following the test is approximately 1 per cent. About one quarter of patients having CVS experience a small amount of vaginal bleeding, usually only a spot or two for one to two days following the procedure.

Diagnostic ultrasound

Diagnostic ultrasound is capable of diagnosing many structural abnormalities during the first half of pregnancy. Many abnormalities may be seen during a scan performed for some other reason whilst others must be looked for specifically. These specific examinations are best undertaken at between 18 to 20 weeks from the commencement of the last menstrual period. A scan undertaken before amniocentesis may be satisfactory in this regard, however the scan performed before chorionic villous sampling is too early in pregnancy to provide information about the normality or otherwise of the fetus.

Fetal blood sampling (FBS)

This involves the removal of a small sample of blood from the baby's umbilical cord at or after 18 weeks. Using local anaesthetic a needle is passed into the uterus and its path is guided by ultrasound. This technique is used in the management of fetal anaemia, investigating possible harmful viral infections and for obtaining fetal blood cells for rapid diagnosis (three to four days) when babies are suspected of having abnormal chromosones.

Some women have more tests than others
▼▼▼

Undoubtedly newer techniques will evolve; however it is important to remember that there is no one test or battery of tests that can tell you if your child is normal. Fortunately the great majority of them are.

AMNIOCENTESIS IN LATE PREGNANCY

In late pregnancy, the test is used in the management of women with Rhesus iso-immunisation and also where there is some doubt as to the duration of the pregnancy. If it is felt that the baby will benefit from delivery, the amniotic fluid can be tested to see whether or not the baby will develop hyaline membrane disease if delivered early (see page 92). If the test shows that there is no danger of this, delivery can go forward as planned; if not, the delivery can be postponed until there is no danger to either the woman or the baby.

The following is a simple method of monitoring the growth rate of a baby. Fundal height should be measured from the fundus of the uterus to the top of the symphysis pubis, with the tape measure lying in contact with the skin of the abdominal wall.

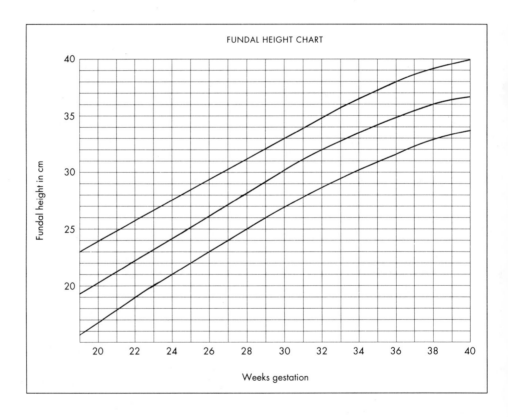

FUNDAL HEIGHT CHART

Fundal height in cm

Weeks gestation

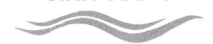

CHAPTER 8

WHEN SHOULD WE GO TO THE HOSPITAL?

The Onset of Labour

THE BODY'S PREPARATION *for* LABOUR

In the last few weeks of pregnancy a variety of things happen in and to the uterus, which finally culminate in the onset of labour.

The Braxton-Hicks contractions of the uterus become stronger and more frequent. These have been occurring in a pattern of every 15 to 20 minutes throughout pregnancy.

The uterus gets ready for labour
▼▼▼

The part of the baby which will be born first, called the presenting part, moves down into the pelvis. This presenting part is usually the baby's head. At the same time, the lower segment of the uterus is thinning out and expanding.

In a woman who has had children, the descent into the pelvis of the presenting part may not occur until labour begins.

The resulting pressure on the cervix may cause it to open or dilate slightly. It is common for the cervix to be 1 to 2 cm dilated before labour begins.

The thick
upper part of
the uterus
does all the
work
▼▼▼

UTERINE CONTRACTIONS

The contractions of true labour may commence suddenly at five to 10 minute intervals and continue, but in some cases they begin gradually at intervals of 15 to 20 minutes and slowly increase in frequency and intensity.

The wall of the uterus is made up of muscle fibres which interlace to form a meshwork of muscle tissue with a small amount of fibrous tissue binding it together. While the muscle cells increase in number during pregnancy they also grow longer and wider. The upper three-quarters of the body of the uterus (the upper uterine segment) is the active contracting part, where all the work is done. Its activity during labour causes the lower portion of the uterus (lower uterine segment) to thin out; it also thins and ultimately dilates the cervix as labour progresses. The muscle cells of the upper segment, like all other muscle cells, have the property of rhythmic contraction. Unlike other cells, however, they can also retract and become shorter after the muscle relaxes. It is the power of retraction that gradually pushes the baby out of the uterus during labour.

No one knows precisely how labour commences. It is probably a complex interplay between hormones and chemicals from the mother and placenta as well as from the baby. Often there is a gradual transition from the Braxton-Hicks contractions into labour contractions. The pattern of regular contractions increasing in

strength, frequency and duration finally makes the woman realise that labour has commenced. As a contraction rises to a peak and then subsides over approximately one minute, discomfort is felt in the lower part of the back passing around both sides of the body to the lower abdomen before fading away. The time to go to hospital is when the contractions have been coming at intervals of 10 minutes or less for one hour. They are not always painful.

Some women complain of backache during the early part of labour. The discomfort is intermittent and if it is due to the onset of labour it will coincide with a hardening of the uterus which can easily be felt by placing the hands on the abdomen. A constant pain in the abdomen or the back, particularly if it is pain associated with hardening or tenderness of the abdomen, may indicate a haemorrhage inside the uterus. This should be reported at once and the woman should go directly to the hospital.

There is a tendency nowadays to stay at home during the early part of the first stage of labour, particularly if it is the first baby. If the woman keeps active, doing light household tasks, cooking or walking, her labour is likely to appear shorter because she is distracted. A phone call to the labour ward at her hospital would reassure her whether it was advisable for her to stay at home for this period. Spending the first few hours of labour moving about, changing positions, and doing stretching exercises is usually more restful than spending the time in the labour ward.

Generally with the first baby, arrival at the labour ward would be desirable when contractions are regular and about five to seven minutes apart.

FALSE LABOUR

Episodes of false labour can occur in the last few weeks of pregnancy. They are more common with second and third babies. In a false labour the pattern of contractions is usually irregular, rarely occurring as often as every 10 minutes. Each contraction may last from 30 seconds to one minute. The active upper part of the uterus tightens and feels hard as the muscle contracts. The feeling is often likened to that of a menstrual cramp or colic, but is often more intense; it is located in the lower part of the abdomen and occasionally low down in the back. False labour does not cause progressive dilation of the cervix.

THE 'SHOW'

Particularly when having a first baby, the onset of labour is not always strictly 'according to the books'. The mother-to-be may have a restless night, followed by a backache during the day, followed by period-like pains which come and go for a few hours, then cease after several hours of sleep. The contractions often begin at approximately 20 or 30 minute intervals, accompanied by a small 'show' of blood and mucus from the vagina. The 'show' may be pink if the blood and mucus are mixed or there may be red streaks of blood on the surface of the mucus. This 'show' should not normally be excessive and the amount of blood and mucus should not require the use of more than one sanitary pad. It is possible to have this show 24 hours or more before any other signs of labour occur.

Bleeding, on the other hand, particularly if it continues, may indicate that part of the placenta has separated from the uterine wall, and for this reason it is important to be seen by the doctor.

RUPTURE *of the* MEMBRANES

The bag of membranes containing the fluid within which the baby lies may rupture, either after labour has commenced or without any other sign of labour. The fluid released by this rupture could be confused with a little gush of urine, accidentally passed, but it is clearer than urine — more like water and without the odour of urine. Once the membranes have ruptured, a small amount of amniotic fluid usually continues to trickle away, and labour usually begins shortly afterwards. It is always wisest to come to the hospital if the membranes have ruptured. If it occurs in the last week or two and labour does not ensue, the doctor may decide it is necessary to induce contractions.

False labour tends to stop and start
▼▼▼

Mucus is squeezed from the cervix as it dilates
▼▼▼

Liquor may appear in a gush or a trickle
▼▼▼

EXPECTED DATE *of* DELIVERY

Women are given a date when they are most likely to expect the onset of labour; it is known as the EDD (expected date of delivery).

About 5 per cent of them come into labour on that day. Some 80 per cent come into labour within 10 days of that date, either before or after, so it is wise to have a bag packed some weeks before your expected date of delivery in case a quick trip to hospital becomes necessary.

ADMISSION *to* HOSPITAL

On arrival at the hospital the first point of contact is the reception desk. As the woman in almost all cases will already have been booked into the hospital, very little paperwork, if any, will need to be completed. However, if the birth is imminent, information can usually be provided by the partner while the woman is taken to the delivery suite, or it can be obtained from the courtesy card which the woman should carry with her. This is the duplicate copy of her prenatal history provided by her doctor or clinic.

Any jewellery will be deposited in a locked cupboard for safekeeping (and a receipt issued); it may be possible to keep rings on, covered with a piece of sticking plaster for safety. In addition, an identity bracelet will be put on the woman's wrist (and also on the baby's wrist as

soon as it is born); these will not be removed until mother and baby leave the hospital.

When the parents come to the delivery suite the sister on duty immediately assesses whether the birth of the baby is imminent. If a drive through heavy traffic has delayed a woman getting to hospital or if she has had one or two babies before, the baby may be ready to be born straight away.

The routine procedure after admission is usually a matter of checking that all is proceeding normally, very like a prenatal visit to the doctor. A specimen of urine is tested, the woman is weighed and she changes into the gown she will wear for her delivery. Some hospitals provide a gown, others suggest that women bring their own nightdress.

Temperature, pulse and blood pressure are checked, the baby's position in the uterus is felt and the baby's heart-beat is counted by listening with a fetal stethoscope. Sometimes the baby's head is far down in the mother's pelvis and regular vaginal examinations are needed to determine the progress of labour.

When constipation has been a problem, it may be necessary for an enema to be given. This helps avoid the expression of bowel motions during delivery of the baby and it may also accelerate labour a little, which is usually welcome. If the labour is advanced and the membranes have ruptured, such treatment is usually not given.

After a shower, the woman leaves the admission area, and with her partner may either sit in the delivery area sitting-room or go directly to a delivery room. This depends on the strength and frequency of her contractions, the stage of labour she has reached, and the facilities available at the hospital she attends.

PRE-TERM LABOUR

A small number of women are admitted to hospital before reaching term but with a labour that is established and cannot be stopped. They will give birth to a baby who is among the 5 to 6 per cent that are born before term. A pre-term baby is one which is born before 37 completed weeks. Such a baby may also be a low-birthweight baby, that is, one that weighs less than 2500 g which is the average weight for a baby at 36 weeks. As well as being smaller than a term baby, a pre-term baby may have immature lungs, making it difficult to breathe without assistance after birth.

In over half the cases there is no cause to be found for the pre-term labour. Factors which may be related to pre-term labour include twins, haemorrhage behind the placenta, excessive amounts of amniotic fluid (poly-hydramnios) and certain fetal abnormalities.

POST-TERM PREGNANCY — GREATER THAN 42 WEEKS

A very small number of pregnancies continue beyond term. In many pregnancies described as post-term, the dates are wrong, the woman having conceived in a long menstrual cycle. This might be her normal cycle or it may be produced by stopping taking the Pill.

The risks associated with real post-maturity are twofold: the baby gets marginally larger, and the supply of oxygen to the baby may decrease. The placenta, which supplies the baby with food and oxygen, is only designed to function properly for about 10 months. Usually the baby is born before the efficiency of the placenta starts to decrease. The risks to the baby increase the further the pregnancy goes overdue so the doctor will consider whether the circumstances require that the birth be induced. If the mother and baby are perfectly normal, all that needs to be done is to see the doctor two or three times weekly to ensure that no problem arises. However, in the presence of raised blood pressure, or where there is evidence of fetal compromise, it may be advisable to induce labour.

INDUCTION *of* LABOUR

When labour is to be induced it is usual for the woman to be admitted to hospital the night before. She is taken to the delivery suite where the usual admission procedures are carried out as described earlier. If the bowel is emptied by a small enema or a suppository, this alone is sometimes sufficient to start labour. Otherwise, the usual method of induction is to

Some babies arrive very early . . .

. . . while others are late

rupture the membranes with a pair of forceps or a special hook, inserted through the cervix. This is no more uncomfortable than an ordinary vaginal examination and labour will usually begin within a few hours as the amniotic fluid trickles away.

If labour does not begin promptly it is usual to give an intravenous drip of saline solution containing syntocinon. This is a synthetic drug which has the same effect of producing regular uterine contractions as the naturally occurring hormone pitocin, which is produced by the pituitary gland. The amount of the drip is slowly increased until labour is established. The drip may have to be continued throughout the whole labour but often it can be stopped and labour continues in a normal fashion.

The above method of induction has a high rate of success provided the cervix is favourable and labour is imminent. Frequently the cervix is unfavourable and in these circumstances, rupturing the membranes is not possible and although intravenous syntocinon will produce uterine contractions, progressive cervical dilatation does not occur. The incidence of caesarean section for failed induction in these circumstances is approximately 50 per cent. Nowadays a hormone called Prostaglandin E_2 (PGE$_2$) is introduced into the upper vagina in the form of a gel. Local absorption results in changes in the cervix and a dose or two some six or so hours apart will frequently convert an unfavourable cervix into one that is favourable, thereby ensuring a successful induction of labour followed by a vaginal delivery.

Induction is performed in the interests of the mother or of the baby
▼▼▼

A special method where doubt exists
▼▼▼

Sometimes labour commences after a dose of PGE$_2$ and its onset is slow, like natural labour and is associated with less need for pain relief than the syntocinon-driven labour. It is believed that this slow onset of labour also permits the baby to adjust to the stress of repeated contractions and lessens the incidence of fetal distress.

Generally women who have an induction of labour are a little more apprehensive than those who do not and may therefore require more relief for pain. If the woman and her partner understand the reason for the induction and have both been involved in the decision to carry it out, as should always be the case, their apprehension will be lessened.

TRIAL *of* LABOUR

A trial of labour simply means trying to achieve a normal vaginal delivery, with provision made for alternative treatment if it becomes clear that this is not possible. This requires that the woman come to the hospital as soon as possible after the onset of labour so that her progress can be carefully monitored.

Women for whom this trial of labour is attempted are very carefully selected as being most likely to be able to have a vaginal delivery even though certain complications exist. These are women who may have had a previous caesarean section or where it is suspected that the woman's pelvis may not be quite large enough to allow the baby's head to descend through it.

During a trial of labour, meticulous attention is given to all observations and most women will deliver normally or at the most have an easy assisted delivery. Often an electrode is attached to the baby's scalp to record the fetal heart rate throughout the labour, and to detect any change that might indicate distress in the baby. Or an external monitor lightly strapped on the abdomen can record the baby's heartbeat by ultrasound. Should the labour progress too slowly or the baby shows signs of distress, the trial of labour can be abandoned and a caesarean section will be performed.

ELECTIVE CAESAREAN SECTION

Some 5 to 10 per cent of women are admitted to hospital knowing that they will not come into labour but will have an elective caesarean section (see Chapter 11: *Another way to have a baby*).

In these cases admission is scheduled for the day before the operation, unless the woman is actually in hospital at the time. The usual time for the operation is a week before the due date to avoid the woman going into labour and endangering herself and the baby. The mother will usually receive intravenous fluids for the first 12 to 24 hours after the operation because of her inability to take adequate fluids and nourishment by mouth.

This chapter would not be complete without mentioning induction of labour or caesarean section performed for convenience. These procedures should be condemned. The only possible exceptions occur where a woman lives a very long distance from the hospital or where previous labours have been exceptionally quick. However, in these situations it may be in the patient's best interest to ensure that she books into the hospital that is closest to her home. Labour should not be induced except for very good obstetric reasons and the most common indication for doing so nowadays is when a pregnancy has been prolonged more than two weeks past the estimated date of delivery for reasons previously outlined. Whenever induction of labour is indicated, both parents should be fully informed of the reasons why it is considered necessary so that they may understand and give an informed consent to the procedure.

A very special method of birth where no doubt exists
▼▼▼

Induction of labour or caesarean section is not an easy way out
▼▼▼

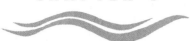

CHAPTER 9

HOW MUCH LONGER, SISTER?

First Stage of Labour and Pain Relief

'Labour' is the word traditionally used to describe the process of giving birth. Although other terms such as 'birthing' and 'birth process' are sometimes used in preference, the word labour is used throughout this and subsequent chapters as it is the name most familiar to people.

The process of labour is usually considered in three stages. The first and longest stage extends from the onset of labour until the cervix is fully open. The second stage follows immediately and ends with the delivery of the baby. The third stage then begins, and lasts until delivery of the placenta and membranes.

> *Contractions start at the top of the uterus*
> ▼▼▼

This chapter deals only with the first stage of labour, although it can be very difficult to establish a clear distinction between the first and second stages.

UTERINE CONTRACTIONS

Each contraction begins near the top of the uterus and spreads downwards in a spiralling fashion until the whole body of the uterus feels hard and tight. The contraction reaches a peak and relaxes gradually, taking as long to fade away as it did to build up.

When relaxed, a pregnant uterus lies moulded against the maternal spine. During a contraction it is lifted forward against the abdominal wall and projects as a hard round lump, particularly in the upper abdomen. With each contraction, a small amount of retraction or shortening of the muscle fibres occurs and this has the effect of pulling up the lower part of the body of the uterus and cervix. As a result, the cervix shortens (takes up) and its opening becomes larger.

During the first stage of labour the cervix can be likened to a barrier: the baby lies behind it, and until the cervix is fully opened, the baby cannot move out of the uterus into the vagina.

Uterine contractions are purely involuntary and vary greatly from one woman to another. As a general rule, the intervals between contractions in the first stage vary from three to six minutes, with each contraction lasting about one minute. As the labour progresses, the contractions occur closer together, last longer and become obviously stronger.

EVENTS *in the* FIRST STAGE *of* LABOUR

The average length of labour in first pregnancies is about 12 hours and in subsequent pregnancies about six hours. The most useful indication of progress is the rate at which the cervix opens up, although obviously the type and pattern of uterine contractions are also important factors.

The cervix is usually 1 to 2 cm open when labour begins. In first labours, the initial opening up of the cervix, known as the latent phase, is slow and may last up to eight hours. This portion of labour is mainly concerned with softening and thinning out the cervix and pulling the cervix up into the lower segment of the uterus, a process described as being somewhat like pulling the sleeve of a sweater over one's fist. At the end of this latent phase, the cervix is only about 4 cm dilated, the size of a 50 cent coin.

Over the next three to four hours a stage of more rapid opening (the active phase) takes place. More

The cervix opens slowly at the beginning of labour

▼▼▼

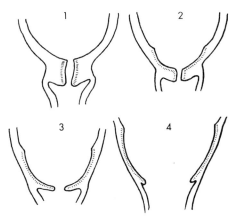

*Dilatation of the cervix
Primigravida*

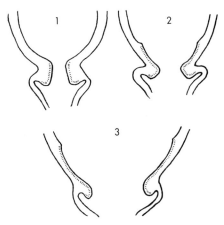

*Dilatation of the cervix
Multipara*

rapidly occurring contractions push the baby's head lower into the pelvis, against the cervix, helping it to open steadily to about 9 cm. Very frequent and strong contractions with little rest between them then follow, finally opening the cervix fully (to a diameter of about 10 cm).

The last part of the first stage of labour is called transition. With second and subsequent babies the latent phase is shorter than in first pregnancies. The active phase lasts much the same length of time.

As the cervix thins out and then starts opening, there is frequently a further slight 'show' of blood and mucus. This is due to the membranes bulging through the cervix and separating from the wall of the lower segment of the uterus. The amount of blood is usually quite small and it may continue to appear from time to time during the latter half of the first stage of labour.

Vaginal examinations are carried out at intervals, in order to determine that labour is progressing normally and to assess how fast the cervix is opening and to ascertain descent of the fetal head.

FIRST STAGE CONTRACTIONS — WHAT THE WOMAN FEELS

Bearing in mind that there are great individual variations, there are some symptoms and feelings during labour which are common to most women.

Many women describe the pain felt during the early part of labour as being mild discomfort and like period pains. A cramping pain which builds up and dies away in time with each contraction of the uterus is felt mainly across the lower abdomen. Sometimes contractions cause an unpleasant backache.

The contractions of the second half of the first stage of labour are probably the most painful that the woman will feel during the whole labour, and as it is too early to 'bear down' (push with her abdominal muscles), it is during this time that she needs most support from her partner and her assistants. The last hour or two of the first stage are associated with frequent strong contractions with little rest between them. It is reassuring to know, however, that progress is ocurring and that the birth is not far away.

Once the cervix is fully opened, it virtually disappears and becomes continuous with the walls of the uterus and vagina. At this stage the woman begins to feel pressure on her bowel. Each contraction can produce a feeling of wanting to hold the breath during the peak of the contraction and bear down. This is a warning that the second stage of labour is near. She is discouraged from bearing down until the cervix is fully dilated, as it may tire her unnessarily; however, if she feels the urge to bear down when there is still a small amount of cervix felt on vaginal examination, the midwife will advise her to breathe quietly with her lips parted during the contractions as this makes it nearly impossible to bear down effectively.

If the membranes have not broken before this stage is reached, they probably will now.

DILATATION OF THE CERVIX — WHAT THE WOMAN FEELS

The woman is not aware of the cervix actually dilating, although she is conscious of the uterus contracting and of a persistent backache. Some women complain of pain over the pubic area which is caused by the baby's head pressing on the cervix or on the joint between the pubic bones. Others notice pain down the inside of both thighs which is related to the stretching of the cervix and pressure on the nerves inside the pelvis.

At the beginning of labour the wall of the cervix is very often about as thick as a little finger, and as well as opening it becomes thinner during the labour. This cannot be felt by the woman and can only be detected by examination. If the cervix was thick and hard at the beginning of labour, real progress has occurred once it begins to soften and thin out, even if it is not dilating as quickly as expected.

AID DURING THE FIRST STAGE OF LABOUR

As has already been mentioned, the first stage of labour is the longest and this particularly applies to the first labour. The expectant woman usually comes to hospital in early labour when contractions are coming at quite long intervals. Time is likely to pass more quickly for her if she can walk around as she has done at home. At this time she rarely feels hungry, but may be quite thirsty. Frequent small amounts of fluids with glucose are quickly digested and give enough energy. By not overloading the

stomach there is less risk of vomiting which can be quite distressing during labour. Sipping iced water or sucking ice fragments is especially helpful if nausea has been a problem, or if the mouth is dry from controlled breathing or from using the nitrous oxide gas (see page 116). Most birth attendants advise against taking solid food once labour is really established, as digestion in the stomach tends to stop once labour begins.

It is important to keep changing position: walking, swaying, showering, massaging, talking and encouraging. Probably most comforting is the presence of a loving and caring partner.

DESCENT OF THE BABY

At the last three or four prenatal visits the midwife/doctor will have checked the position of the baby in the uterus, noting how much of the baby's head can be felt through the abdomen.

Towards the end of pregnancy, the baby's head begins to settle lower

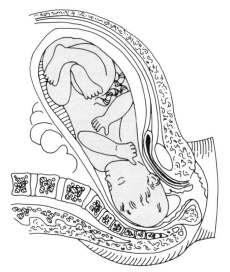

First stage of labour: cervix half dilated

You can't feel the cervix opening
▼▼▼

Simple things often help.
▼▼▼

How the baby's head moves through the pelvis
▼▼▼

in the pelvis and becomes more difficult to feel. The woman may feel the baby's head descending but this is not always the case, as the descent is normally slow, particularly for a first baby. As the head presses down on her bladder she often complains of passing urine more frequently. One consolation is that the baby is probably not pressing on her stomach so severely or kicking so strongly as there is now not enough room for it to do so.

During labour the midwife follows the descent of the baby's head by feeling the abdomen. When only a small amount of the baby's head can be felt, it means that the widest part of the head is deeply settled into the pelvis and is pressing against the cervix. The baby's head is engaged.

The baby seems to know that it may be a tight fit and bends the chin firmly on the chest to make the smallest part of the head descend first through the birth canal. When the baby's head is a little deflexed (bent slightly backwards), resulting in a wider part of the head trying to come through the birth canal first, the progress is slower. This is often the case when the baby is facing forwards in the uterus rather than backwards. This is known as an occipito-posterior position of the head. The baby's head usually turns around as it moves downwards so that the 'pointiest' part of the head is distending the birth canal. Sometimes the baby remains 'posterior' and is delivered as such. This is not abnormal. The position of the baby's head is not luck but a result of the taking up of the best available space in the pelvis.

MOULDING AND CAPUT

During labour the baby's head is moulded to the shape of the birth canal. The soft skull bones partly overlap each other to allow the shape of the baby's head to alter from a round shape to an elongated shape as labour progresses. This moulding enables the baby's head to be as small as possible, so that the birth canal will not have to stretch unreasonably. The shape of the baby's head usually returns to normal within a few hours after birth, although it may take up to 48 hours.

Caput is a term used to describe a small part of the baby's scalp which has swollen during labour. This swelling consists of waterlogged tissue caused by pressure against the cervix and for that reason it is like a small, round lump on the head. It has no ill effects and it also disappears after several days.

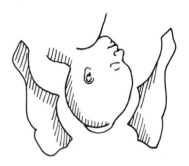

Head moulding and formation of caput

MONITORING *the* LABOUR

The term 'monitoring' means to keep a close watch on something. Both mother and baby are monitored during the course of labour by the midwife. In some labours the baby may be more closely monitored by electronic means.

Apart from any special needs, the woman has her pulse, blood pressure and temperature taken at approximately hourly intervals during labour. Any urine that is passed is tested for sugar and protein as well as substances called ketones whose presence would indicate that she is low on blood sugar and dehydrated. Vaginal examinations are performed at intervals of two to four hours to assess the progress of labour.

The baby's condition is checked by listening to and counting its heart rate, and also by making sure that any amniotic fluid that is passed from the vagina does not contain a substance called meconium. Meconium is the normal dark green contents of the baby's bowel. It is common for meconium to be present in the amniotic fluid at the end of pregnancy. Sometimes, however, this can indicate fetal distress and so fetal monitoring is always advised.

The baby's heart rate during labour varies from 120 to 160 beats per minute. As the cervix nears full dilatation during the second stage, the stronger contractions cause pressure on the baby's head and it is normal at this stage for its heart rate to slow down at the height of a contraction and to return to normal as the contraction eases off. However, any slowing of the baby's heart rate during the early part of labour is unusual, and if it is noticed the baby's heart rate will be monitored by means of a fetal monitor.

Each time the uterus contracts, the pressure inside it increases. During strong contractions the blood flow through the placenta is decreased and this cuts down the oxygen supply to the baby. Normally this has little effect on the baby who can easily withstand such short periods of oxygen deprivation. However, some babies are not able to cope as well as others and their heart rate slows with contractions in the early part of labour.

Monitoring of the baby may be done externally or internally. In external monitoring, an ultrasound disc is strapped to the maternal abdomen, and when attached to a fetal monitor, it provides a record of the baby's heart rate. Another disc is placed higher on the maternal abdomen to record the uterine contractions. In this way the response of the baby's heart rate to each contraction can be accurately assessed. This form of monitoring may be uncomfortable for the woman, and if she changes position, the positions of the two discs have to be changed.

More accurate information, however, can be obtained by internal monitoring where a thin tube is inserted into the mother's uterus to measure the pressure changes and a small electrode is attached to the baby's head to record its heart rate. As the woman has nothing strapped to her abdomen, she is more comfortable and can move around in bed more freely, although she is unable to walk around.

Machines can be used to help check the baby's condition

▼▼▼

FETAL DISTRESS

This is the term used to describe a number of situations that can arise during labour which may indicate that the baby is in danger of damage or, in extreme cases, of dying.

If the baby's heart rate rises above 160 or falls below 120 or is slow to return to its normal rate following a uterine contraction, it is common to monitor the baby electronically. If the heart rate is persistently slow to recover, it is a sign that for some reason or another the baby is not receiving the optimal supply of oxygen. A small amount of blood can then be obtained from the baby's scalp, and the amount of oxygen in and the acidity of this blood are measured. If there is adequate oxygen in the sample and its acidity is normal, labour is allowed to continue although the test will need to be repeated within an hour or so.

If the oxygen content of the sample is low or there is a high level of acidity, quick delivery of the baby will be considered. If this happens early in the first stage of labour, it will mean delivery by caesarean section. If it occurs at the end of the first stage of labour, it may be possible to wait until the second stage commences and then deliver the baby with forceps.

It has been argued that the use of monitors has increased the incidence of caesarean section, but where reliable statistics are obtained and interpreted accurately, this has been shown not to be the case.

Approximately 90 per cent of pregnancies are normal and remain so during labour. Careful observation during labour enables any

abnormalities to be identified at an early stage and treated correctly.

CAUSES *of a* LONG FIRST STAGE *of* LABOUR

If a labour is prolonged, assistance may be considered. Continued progress with adequate uterine power must be demonstrated in successful labour.

The commonest cause of a long first stage of labour is failure of the uterus to contract efficiently. This is most common in a first labour. The contractions are not only weak and of short duration but also tend to be irregular and infrequent. It rarely occurs in subsequent pregnancies. When uterine contractions occur in this pattern, the cervix opens only slowly, which is disappointing. This disappointment, in addition to the fact that she is unable to rest adequately can lead to a deterioration in the woman's morale, despite the best emotional support.

Good support, encouragement, relaxation and pain relief will reduce anxiety, the cause of excessive production of adrenalin and other factors that may make the uterine muscle too irritable and incoordinate. Augmentation of the contractions with syntocinon in the vein may be used to help increase the strength of contractions.

Another cause of a long first stage of labour is disproportion. This is when the baby is too big to go through the mother's pelvis or the pelvis is too small to allow even a normal-sized baby to pass through it.

Disproportion may be either absolute (the baby's head is too big for the pelvis), in which case it calls for a caesarean section, or relative which is mainly due to a faulty position of the baby, which hopefully will correct itself as labour progresses.

The commonest fault in the position of the baby occurs when the baby is facing forwards — an occipito-posterior or, simply, a 'posterior'. While progress occurs, even if only slowly, there is no need to interfere. However, if over a period of three to four hours there is no progress in opening of the cervix or descent of the baby's head through the pelvis, a caesarean birth may be considered, even if the uterus is contracting efficiently.

PAIN *and* PAIN RELIEF

It is interesting to remember that when John Snow administered chloroform to Queen Victoria over 100 years ago for the birth of one of her children, he was looked upon by women as a saviour. However, he was condemned by other people, particularly churchmen, for interfering in what they believed was meant to be a painful process!

Many women approaching the time of giving birth are still very afraid that they may be going to experience pain beyond their endurance. There are many sources of the belief that childbirth is inevitably associated with prolonged agony; apart from popular ill-informed mythology, scenes from old films such as *Gone with the Wind* and *Anna Karenina* do nothing to provide reassurance. Happily, the unfortunate heroines of those classics are not typical obstetric patients, and furthermore they would certainly not experience the same misery today.

It is impossible to predict accurately how labour will affect each woman. The discomforts of labour vary greatly from woman to woman, from labour to labour in the same woman, and from stage to stage of each labour. For this reason it is impossible to generalise about pain and pain relief; each woman has her own individual needs.

About 10 per cent of all women have a relatively easy labour which gives them intense satisfaction. Many factors are involved in this happy outcome including: baby size, pelvis shape and position of baby in the pelvis. Uterine contractions which are well coordinated and efficient will help to assure an even progression of labour. Finally, those areas of the woman's anatomy that have to be widely stretched during delivery must be pliable. These women do not need much help from pain-relieving agents. However, the majority of women in labour will experience discomfort to a degree which could be extremely distressing if help were not available.

It frequently comes as a surprise to women in labour to discover how severe the pain can be when the uterus is contracting strongly. It should be remembered that the uterus is a very strong muscular organ. When its muscles contract, a lot of force is being exerted on the

'Posterior' labours are slower

▼▼▼

Contractions can be painful

▼▼▼

*Sensations
are different
in the second
stage*

▼▼▼

*There is no
set routine*

▼▼▼

*Fear causes
tension,
causing pain*

▼▼▼

*Knowing
about labour
can help*

▼▼▼

*Distraction
can block
pain*

▼▼▼

cervix in order to open it up. It is this pressure on and stretching of the cervix which causes most of the unpleasant sensations of the first stage of labour. The severity of the pain starts as a moderate but quite tolerable discomfort in the early stages of labour, becoming more severe as the strength and frequency of contractions build up. If for some reason the cervix is slow to open, the woman may become distressed because she is discouraged by the apparent lack of progress.

The pain of the second stage is less distressing. As the baby's head starts to descend little by little, stretching the tissues of the vagina and surrounding muscles, the sensation is one of pressure on this area. Almost all women who reach this second stage with few or no drugs, are able to deliver their babies with little or no extra pain relief. The bearing down required in the second stage is often hard physical work. Some women find that it helps to make a lot of noise as they push. Despite appearances to the contrary, the second stage is less distressing and more satisfying than the last part of the first stage.

There are three main methods currently used for relieving labour pains. A woman may use relaxation techniques and distraction procedures known under the general name of psychoprophylaxis (literally, prevention through the power of the mind), which can be learnt in prenatal classes. Or she may choose a variety of sedative and analgesic drugs as and when she needs them. Or she may choose to have a completely painless labour by having

a local anaesthetic injection known as a lumbar epidural block. Sometimes all three techniques are used in the course of one labour: a woman starts with psychoprophylaxis, later requires some sedation, and finally has an epidural block.

PSYCHO-PHYSICAL PREPARATION FOR LABOUR

Over the last 50 years there have been many attempts to alleviate the pain of labour by education, explanation and prenatal training. A method known as 'Natural Childbirth' was introduced in the 1930s by Dr Grantly Dick Read. He believed that pain was largely a result of abnormal emotional tension which was caused by fear, and that if we get rid of this fear and encourage a relaxed and peaceful state of mind, the pain of labour will largely be eliminated. This has proven to be partially correct.

Unfortunately, too much was expected of Natural Childbirth, and many women were grievously disillusioned and disappointed when, despite their most earnest endeavours, they suffered a great deal of pain. However, it did spark an interest in the psychological preparation for labour which has developed and expanded, particularly in the last 20 years, and is now an important aspect of the prenatal period.

Education about the process of labour and delivery is available to all pregnant women and their partners. A sound basic understanding of what is to take place always reduces anxiety and apprehension. All hospitals offer evening lectures given by hospital staff, and there are also enthusiastic lay organisations which provide instruction classes, books and pamphlets on all aspects of pregnancy and childbirth. The aim of education is for couples to come to see childbirth as a normal, natural process, to understand it and to participate actively in it.

At the classes, exercises designed by physiotherapists to encourage relaxation during labour are taught. The exercises include breathing patterns to be used during contractions. Relaxation and breathing exercises reduce muscular tension and it is probable that these exercises also act as a form of distraction therapy, giving the labouring woman something to concentrate on apart from her discomfort.

The most highly developed regimen of prenatal training was developed by Russian and French doctors who gave it the name psychoprophylaxis. This is taught both by lay organisations, particularly the Childbirth Education Association, and many hospital-based physiotherapy departments. It is practised with great enthusiasm by a very large number of women who are anxious to have as normal a delivery as possible and avoid the use of drugs as much as possible. When properly trained in the technique, a woman in labour will use specific breathing patterns in response to the contractions: as the contractions increase in intensity she alters her breathing patterns accordingly.

Psychoprophylaxis also trains a woman not to tense her muscles as a contraction builds up, but deliberately to relax her limbs and the muscles of her pelvic floor. This is not too difficult in the early stages, but as labour progresses it requires a high degree of control. She is shown a variety of positions and postures that she can adopt during labour.

An important feature of the psychoprophylaxis technique is the assistance of the partner or other supporter who learns about the method, attends as many of the training sessions as possible and helps with the home practice. The partner supplies support and encouragement during labour and this joint participation in the event of childbirth helps to enhance the couple's relationship and their bonds with their child.

It is difficult to assess how successful any particular method of training for childbirth is, as some 10 per cent of women having their first baby, and considerably more with subsequent pregnancies, have a virtually painless first stage of labour and a relatively short second stage irrespective of whether or not they have had any special prenatal preparation. However, surveys show that about 20 per cent of women having their first baby feel that psychoprophylaxis helped them considerably (this group of women naturally includes the 10 per cent who would have had a relatively easy time of it anyway, with or without preparation).

Another 60 to 70 per cent feel the programme benefited them to a satisfactory degree. These women may or may not have needed some extra assistance in the form of analgesic drugs.

This leaves 10 to 15 per cent of women whose first labours are so

The stimulus determines the response
▼▼▼

Relaxing is not always easy
▼▼▼

A support person is important
▼▼▼

abnormally painful and incoordinate, that nothing short of the complete pain relief offered by an epidural block (see page 117) makes the event bearable. In subsequent pregnancies many of these women are surprised to find their labour is so easy that by the time they ask for pain relief, the baby is about to be born.

In any event, it is important that any woman who needs to ask for medication should never think that she has failed or feel guilty in any way. It is both foolish and futile to battle on becoming more and more distressed when safe and effective relief is available for the asking.

While nobody would claim that psycho-physical methods of preparation are completely successful in all cases, there is no doubt that they do reduce the total amount of analgesic drugs required.

ANALGESIA

Analgesia is a term used to describe the relief of pain by any means without loss of consciousness, and analgesia may be offered to a woman in labour according to her needs and desires.

Narcotic drugs

These are used widely to relieve labour pain. They have to be given by injection to ensure proper absorption into the blood stream. The most commonly used narcotic is pethidine, which is effective as a painkiller for two or three hours. Apart from relieving pain, it also causes a light-headed feeling, some drowsiness, and sometimes dizziness. As its effect wears off, the injection can be repeated, provided delivery is not

expected within the next four hours, as the drug does pass across the placenta and may cause the baby to be a bit drowsy at birth and therefore reluctant to breathe deeply. If this should happen, an antidote can be injected into the umbilical cord after the baby is delivered, quickly reversing the effects of the pethidine.

Pethidine is used very commonly and is recognised to be safe and reasonably effective in reducing the severity of the pain of contractions. However, in many cases it is found that as labour progresses, something else is needed as well as pethidine. When this stage is reached the patient is offered nitrous oxide.

Nitrous oxide

Nitrous oxide has been a great stand-by in labour wards for 50 years. It is the old 'laughing gas' and is particularly safe for mother and child. This form of analgesia is administered by the woman herself through a mask, whenever she feels the need for pain relief. She inhales as each contraction begins and lays the mask aside between contractions.

Nitrous oxide is mixed with oxygen. The usual mixture contains 30 to 50 per cent oxygen, which compares favourably with the air we are all breathing which contains only 20 per cent oxygen. So mother and baby run no risk of suffering from lack of oxygen. The concentration of gas used is adjusted by the midwife, who also teaches the mother how to hold the mask on her face and use it correctly. Nitrous oxide has no effect at all on the state of the baby at birth, and disappears immediately from the woman's body as soon as she stops breathing it.

Nitrous oxide has a slight rubbery smell, which a few people object to, and it also causes a sensation of floating and light-headedness.

Like all other analgesic drugs, nitrous oxide has to get to the brain to have its effect, and this takes about 20 seconds from the beginning of the inhalation. If it is not inhaled until a contraction is reaching its peak it will be too late for it to help. It is most important to start breathing the gas at the very beginning of a contraction, if not slightly before, so that there is a useful amount built up in the brain by the time the contraction reaches its painful peak.

More than half of all women find that a combination of pethidine and nitrous oxide provides an adequate degree of analgesia during labour. For the others it is necessary to turn to a more complicated technique known as an epidural block.

Epidural anaesthesia

Epidurals are so called after an anatomical space of that name within the spinal canal. If a local anaesthetic solution is injected into that space low down in the back, it will temporarily block the transmission of pain sensation along the nerve roots that pass through the epidural space on the way to the spinal cord. This technique of analgesia has been known since the beginning of the century and has been used increasingly over the last 30 years for a wide variety of surgical operations on the lower half of the body and, in lesser strengths, in obstetrics. It is now an accepted technique in all labour wards and is certainly the most effective method of controlling severe pain during labour and delivery.

When an epidural block is used for pain relief it is usually inserted in the first stage of labour when the cervix is about half dilated, but there is no reason why it should not be done earlier if necessary. The decision to have an epidural is made by the woman in discussion with the obstetrician, midwife and anaesthetist. It would never be done on an unwilling patient; most epidurals are given in response to the patient's direct request.

An anaesthetist performs an epidural block. It takes about five minutes, during which time the woman lies on her side curled up as much as possible to open up the spaces between the vertebrae.

The insertion of the needle is no more painful than an ordinary injection, and once the injection has been made, relief from labour pain is noticed after about three minutes. The numbness gradually sets in over the lower half of the body and legs. The degree of numbness varies between women. The legs feel heavy and warm and cannot easily be moved. Contractions and, during the second stage, pressure from the baby's head may still be felt, but there is no pain.

A fine plastic tube (an epidural catheter) is usually inserted into the epidural space when the first injection is made. This allows for 'top-ups' to maintain the analgesia as long as necessary. The effect of each dose lasts for about three hours.

There is no doubt that the use of epidurals has transformed the attitudes and experiences of many thousands of women in labour. For the first time any woman can have

Epidurals are a great help if the labour is long
▼▼▼

The injection does not have to be repeated
▼▼▼

complete relief from pain without being unconscious and without endangering her baby.

There are, however, some disadvantages to this method of pain relief of which everyone should be aware. It is a far more complicated technique than is the use of pethidine and nitrous oxide. Also, an epidural may remove the urge to bear down, so in a number of cases the baby cannot be pushed out by the mother's efforts, and a simple forceps delivery or ventouse (a suction cup), is necessary. In skilled hands this does no harm at all to the baby. Some women are disappointed by this form of delivery. (See Chapter 10: *Is it all right if I push?*)

Occasionally, in about one in 200 cases, the epidural needle goes in slightly too far, making a hole in the dura, which is a fibrous sheath surrounding the spinal cord. The hole is itself not important, but the resultant loss of fluid from inside the dura may cause a headache which may last up to a week.

Backaches are quite common in the early days after labour. However, they have not been found to be any more common among women who have had an epidural than in those who have had other forms of pain relief or none at all.

Some patients are concerned that there may be a danger of permanent paralysis or nerve injury of some sort. Such a complication is extraordinarily rare, less than one in 100 000 cases.

An epidural block is by far the most effective means of relieving severe labour pains, but it must always be used with great discretion

and only when it is clearly necessary. The woman is usually the best judge of when this form of analgesia should be used. She can at any time discuss this and other methods of pain relief with her doctor and the midwives.

As with other forms of analgesia, it is mostly women having their first baby who find the greatest need for epidurals. Subsequent labours tend to be much quicker and less distressing than the first one and a woman need not request an epidural just because she had one for the delivery of her first baby. She should try the simpler methods first as she may find that they are quite adequate this time.

PUDENDAL BLOCK

This is a method of using local anaesthetic just before delivery. It requires less expertise than an epidural and affects only the perineum (the area between the vaginal opening and the anus) and lower part of the vagina. The local anaesthetic is injected by the obstetrician through each side wall of the vagina, around the pudendal nerves which carry pain sensations from that area. It does not lessen the pain of uterine contractions, but does allow an episiotomy and even a simple forceps delivery to be done almost painlessly.

GENERAL ANAESTHESIA

While analgesia involves relieving pain while the patient remains awake, general anaesthesia renders the patient completely unconscious. Since epidural analgesia has become freely available, the use of general anaesthesia has declined dramatically. There are still a few situations when a general anaesthetic may have to be performed urgently in the labour ward.

The most common reason for its use is the need to remove by hand a placenta that refuses to leave the uterus after the baby has been born. For this to be done it may be necessary to relax a firmly contracted uterus, and a general anaesthetic is the only reliable method of ensuring relaxation.

Another occasion when a general anaesthetic may be necessary is at the delivery of a second twin. It is quite common for the second twin to get itself into an awkward position, which the obstetrician has to correct while it is still in the uterus before delivery can take place. Again, a relaxed uterus is required, and a general anaesthetic rather than an epidural block is needed.

As far as the patient is concerned, a general anaesthetic means instant sleep after a simple intravenous injection. Apart from the disappointment of not being awake to welcome her baby, any patient having a general anaesthetic is exposed to some real hazards and disadvantages; because of these,

general anaesthesia is used only when it is absolutely necessary. There is usually no hazard to the baby, though he or she may be sleepy.

HYPNOSIS

A hypnotic trance can provide enough maternal analgesia for drugs not to be needed. It does not affect the baby and it has been claimed to shorten labour. Hypnosis sounds an ideal method of relieving labour pain, but there are some enormous obstacles to the possibility of using it for large numbers of women. A long series of conditioning sessions with the hypnotist is necessary to prepare a patient for hypnosis, and only a small proportion of women are able to become fully conditioned; and for some the method may fail during labour.

ACUPUNCTURE

This method of producing analgesia has also proved disappointing. It has proved quite inadequate in a large number of cases, making it unacceptable for widespread use in this country. This may well be because our culture has not prepared us to accept it.

General anaesthetics are less common nowadays
▼▼▼

Other methods of pain relief may be used
▼▼▼

CHAPTER 10

IS IT ALL RIGHT IF I PUSH?

Second and Third Stages of Labour

The regular uterine contractions of the first stage of labour have pushed the baby downwards into the pelvis, thinned out the lower segment of the uterus and the cervix, and then pulled the dilating cervix upwards over the baby's head. This means that the head is now in the upper part of the vagina.

This chapter is concerned with the second and third stages of labour which are the birth of the baby and the delivery of the placenta and membranes.

Second stage is a relief
▼▼▼

SECOND STAGE: DELIVERY *of* *the* BABY

Most women find it a wonderful relief to know they are in second stage labour and that their baby is to be born soon, and for many the birth of the baby is a truly enjoyable experience. A prerequisite to this enjoyment is a gentle assistant to help the mother give birth. This assistant is usually either a midwife or the doctor who has been taking care of the woman throughout her pregnancy. Also likely to be assisting at the birth will be a trainee nurse and, if the delivery is taking place in a teaching hospital, there may be a medical student. The partner completes the team of helpers.

POSITIONS *for* DELIVERY

Childbirth that is as natural as possible should be the goal of all involved — the woman, midwife, doctor and partner. The first baby takes the longest to push into the world and so it should be expected that the first labour is the most difficult. A lot of determination by the labouring woman and strong support by her attendants, is required. Of course it is not always possible to achieve natural childbirth but it is worth a good try.

The strong contractions of second stage labour can be overwhelming to both the woman and her partner. Keeping active and changing positions at this time seems to help psychologically, as the woman feels less helpless. It is a good idea to use gravity forces to aid the expulsion of the baby. This includes a multitude of positions both on and off a bed, most with the help of a partner. Very little equipment is needed for an active second stage — a bean bag, pillows, a medium height chair. The woman needs to try various positions to decide which suits her best. It is

important to have a mirror available for the woman to glimpse her baby's head as soon as it is visible — she can really believe her labour has nearly ended.

The following positions have been found helpful during the second stage.

STANDING

Facing partner with arms around the neck — allowing the knees to bend and feet apart. In between contractions, 'pelvic rocking', a circular movement of the hips, keeps this position 'fluid'. This position makes good use of gravity, but can be tiring — variation is necessary.

During labour, changing positions helps
▼▼▼

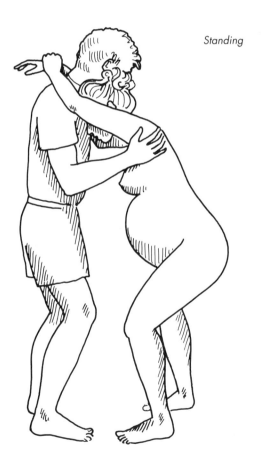

Standing

SQUATTING

The partner sits on a chair, the woman squatting on the floor in front of him — leaning her back against him as he supports her. This is a good position for delivery as well — especially if the woman leans back far enough for her birth attendant to see the advancing baby's head and assess the perineal stretching. This is necessary, so the woman can be instructed to control, by her breathing, the gentle expulsion of the head. The disadvantage is that prolonged squatting may cause a swelling of the perineum, which does not stretch as well.

SITTING

Advantages for the position both for 'pushing down' and delivery is that a bean bag can be punched into shape to fit into the woman's back, and is a good. She can also rest her head back between contractions. An attendant can hold a mirror in the sitting position, as she pulls back on her knees during contractions to complement the natural curve of the birth canal.

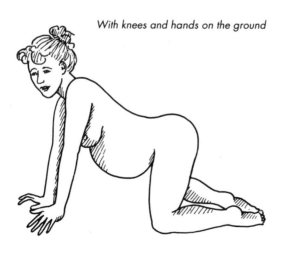

With knees and hands on the ground

To summarise, the woman and her partner should experiment with positions in labour to find one which is most suitable and comfortable. Individuals vary so much in their needs and preferences, and no position should be held for long periods. Continued support and encouragement is the key to success with emphasis on progress not pain.

LENGTH OF THE SECOND STAGE OF LABOUR

Unlike the first stage where the duration varies enormously between women, the second stage runs a more definite, predictable course. With first labours it is likely to last between 30 minutes and a couple of hours, and with the second and subsequent labours it may be as short as 10 to 20 minutes. A second stage longer than two hours is associated with a faulty position of the baby's head such as an occipito-posterior. Few attendants would allow the second stage to proceed for longer than two hours without identifying the cause of the delay and suggesting appropriate management.

SECOND STAGE UTERINE CONTRACTIONS

The contractions of the second stage of labour are more powerful than those of the first stage. They also occur closer together, last longer, but are no more painful than first stage contractions. As the baby's head is moved down into the vagina by each contraction, it produces pressure on the rectum, the lower part of the vagina and the pelvic floor muscles.

This leads to an involuntary bearing down effort in which the throat is closed off, and the breath is held. The muscles of the chest wall and abdomen then contract strongly in an attempt to push the baby out.

EVENTS OF THE SECOND STAGE OF LABOUR

The second stage of labour begins once the cervix is fully dilated. The desire to bear down just before full dilatation can be very strong sometimes. A vaginal examination by the midwife quickly determines if the second stage has indeed begun, for the cervix will then have disappeared above the baby's head, becoming continuous with the walls of the uterus and vagina.

In the early part of labour, the baby's head will usually have entered the pelvis in a transverse position, that is, facing to one side or other, because in this position it lies in the largest diameter of the pelvis. Now, however, at about the time of full dilatation of the cervix and as the baby's head is being pushed further

down in the pelvis, it begins to turn, so that it ends up facing backwards. It does so because of changes in the shape of the pelvis (the available space for the head is now circular rather than oval) and because of the slope of the pelvic floor. The muscle which forms the pelvic floor, the levator ani, acts as a sloping gutter directed downwards and forwards towards the outlet of the pelvis.

If the baby's head is well flexed (tucked in with chin on chest), the first part of it to reach the pelvic floor is the back portion (the occiput). When the head turns, this part comes to lie behind the pubic bone. This position of the head is described as occipito-anterior and is the best position for delivery. The expulsive contractions of the second stage of labour then allow the head to be born facing the mother's back in the widest diameter of the outlet of the pelvis.

The vagina offers similar resistance to the descent of the head as the cervix did but now is the time when active bearing down during each uterine contraction can help

It's hard not to push too soon
▼▼▼

The baby's head turns in the mother's pelvis
▼▼▼

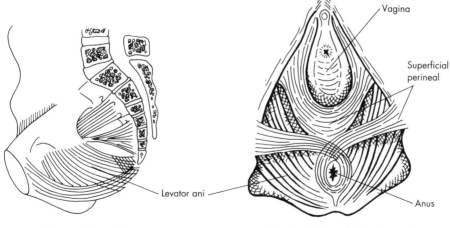

Lateral view of the pelvis, showing muscles of the side wall of the pelvis

Muscles of the pelvis (perineum)

Vagina

Superficial perineal

Levator ani

Anus

with the delivery. However, in the early part of the second stage it is often better to let the contractions do most of the work and quietly bring the baby down on to the pelvic floor.

As the baby's head descends into the pelvis the organs already there are pushed aside. The bladder in front is pulled upwards by the rising cervix and becomes an abdominal organ. In the back part of the pelvis the lower bowel and anus are pushed downwards and backwards and any faeces in the anal canal will be passed at this time. The pelvic floor muscles are pushed downwards and sideways to allow the baby's head to come through the pelvic floor. Pressure on the pelvic floor muscles and rectum give the desire to push.

Some women find second stage labour absolutely terrifying. A sensation of intense pressure of the baby's head on the bowel and a feeling of the body splitting down the middle can be very frightening. Women who have had epidurals can deliver their baby by their own expulsive efforts, though sometimes a simple lift-out forceps delivery may be necessary as the epidural may remove the urge to bear down.

What the woman feels as she is bearing down in childbirth is the extreme stretching of the perineum to allow the baby's head to be born. The vagina is very elastic and stretches easily but the opening of the vagina and the perineal muscles sometimes sustain a tear. After the baby is born, the vagina reverts to almost normal.

The mother finds the bearing down efforts of the second stage of labour quite tiring; no wonder it has been called 'hard labour'. She has

The vagina is very distensible
▼▼▼

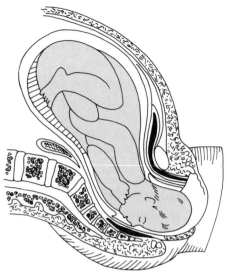

Second stage of labour
Head in view

about two minutes rest between contractions, and should use this time to relax as much as possible.

When the baby's head can be seen and it is starting to distend the vaginal opening, there is a need to push. This should be synchronised with each contraction until the head stays in view between contractions, when it is said to be 'crowned'. By the woman using her muscles to hold the head at the vaginal entrance when she takes a breath, a little advance is made each time.

The pushing stage is completed when the baby's head does not retreat between contractions. Now steady pressure instead of pushing is needed. Usually at this point she is asked to stop bearing down, and to allow only the contractions to push the baby into the world. She will still want to push but can avoid doing so by panting gently. In this way the birth of the baby's head is more gentle and controlled, and in most cases allows the stretched skin around the vaginal opening to continue stretching slowly without tearing.

When the head is born, there is an immediate feeling of relief and relaxation until the next contraction commences.

Even until recently women have been told to push really hard from the beginning of the second stage, before the head has descended or even before it has rotated. This tends to be very tiring for most women and probably does not really shorten the second stage. The baby will be born without this extreme degree of effort. With a little patience on the part of all concerned, most babies are born surprisingly easily.

The attendants wipe any mucus or blood from the baby's eyes, which are usually still closed at this time, and gently suck any mucus or liquor from the mouth and nose using a soft plastic catheter attached to a suction apparatus. While the shoulders and trunk are still in the birth canal the baby does not breathe. The umbilical cord is still providing the baby with oxygen via the placenta, so it is usual to check that the cord is not around the neck. If it is lying loosely around the neck it can be slipped over the head, but if there are several loops or if it appears to be tight, the cord may need to be clamped and cut before the shoulders are born.

The next contraction, aided by a final bearing down effort, delivers the rest of the baby. The midwife holds the baby head-downwards with the feet in right hand while supporting the head with the left. The baby is placed on the mother's abdomen while still attached to the placenta by

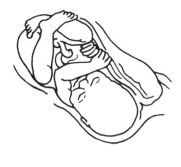
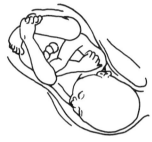
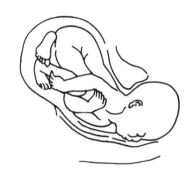
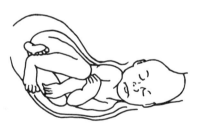

Descent and rotation of the head

the umbilical cord. The cord is then clamped and cut, and the baby loosely wrapped to dry off the wet skin and avoid chilling.

The exhilaration that the parents feel at the birth of their baby, at last, after nine long months and such hard work during labour, is not likely to be forgotten!

FIRST FEW MINUTES AFTER DELIVERY

Many mothers want to put the baby to their breast as soon as possible. Some just like to hold the baby close. Others prefer to see their baby after being cleaned a little by the nurse. Parents should hold their baby as soon as possible after the delivery, but also remember that there is much more involved in bonding than the first minutes of life or the brief time spent in hospital.

At delivery a baby's body must undergo radical changes to adapt from an existence dependent upon the placenta and mother to a more self-reliant state. In the first few minutes after birth, the most important changes occur in the lungs and the blood circulation.

While in the uterus, the lungs are not used for breathing. The placenta absorbs all the oxygen needed from the maternal circulation and eliminates carbon dioxide. The lungs are filled with watery lung fluid and only enough blood circulates through them to enable them to grow and develop.

Delivery changes this situation. Firstly, the pressure of the birth canal on the chest squeezes out much of the lung fluid. This water may be seen running out of the baby's mouth when the head is born. (A soft tube or catheter is usually used to suck the throat and mouth clear at this time.) Within seconds of the rest of the body being delivered, the baby takes the first breath. The remainder of the lung fluid is then rapidly absorbed into the baby's circulation as the lungs become filled with air.

The heart responds to the expansion of the chest with air by re-directing blood away from the placenta to the lungs so that oxygen can be absorbed. The circulation is now completely changed from a single pump system, which sent the blood from the placenta to the body and back to the placenta, to a double pump system which sends half of the blood to the lungs to collect oxygen and sends the other half, which has returned from the lungs, out to the body.

Cord clamping

There has been some debate about the best time to clamp the cord after delivery: straightaway or after it has ceased to pulsate. Certainly the last word has not been said in this argument, but more and more data has accumulated that shows that clamping the cord early (about 10 seconds after birth) seems to produce babies who are more alert, sleep and feed better and generally adapt slightly more quickly to life outside the womb than those whose cords are not clamped immediately. For most babies, though, it is probably not critical either way.

Resuscitation

The vast majority of babies take their first breath and start to cry straight after delivery. There is usually no need to encourage them in any way, and certainly the days of a resounding smack on the bottom are over. Occasionally, for instance after a difficult or prolonged labour, the baby may require some help to start breathing. Using a specially designed 'bag and mask', his chest is inflated with a mixture of oxygen and air and usually this is enough to start things going. The need for this in no way implies that the baby has suffered from lack of oxygen or that trouble

---

Many changes occur in the baby immediately after it is born

▼▼▼

Cord clamping early or late?

▼▼▼

may lie ahead for that baby. A baby's metabolism, and especially his brain metabolism, has been provided with the ability to withstand oxygen deprivation for quite long periods of time without harm.

Some people assume that the baby's first cry represents anguish on the part of the newborn baby and believe that methods should be adopted to decrease the likelihood of the baby crying after the first breath. However, there is no evidence at all that crying at birth represents a less than ideal situation or that an effort to stop it occurring benefits the baby in any way. Indeed, vigorous crying movements probably help the lung fluid to drain out and to establish a good breathing pattern.

Loving and nurturing

It has been noted that soon after delivery, though mother and baby may be physically very tired, both are unusually alert. When put together they seek and maintain eye contact for long periods of time. Mothers stroke their babies and coo words in a high voice, all the time gazing into the baby's eyes and baby gazes fixedly back.

Curiously, this 'face-searching' reflex in the baby tends to diminish markedly after a few hours and does not return as powerfully until several weeks have passed. Like everything else in nature, this gazing reflex has a function. Eye contact evokes very strong maternal feelings, and thus is part of the survival apparatus of the newborn: baby can make mother love and therefore protect him or her!

This initial bonding blends in with the more complex, longterm attachment which is the deep durable love which grows between a mother and her baby. After the initial encounter, mothers grow more attached to their infants each day by touching and feeding them and by looking after all their needs. Mothers feel the impact of maternal feelings in different ways; some attach powerfully on immediate contact, others take longer and grow to love their infants over days and weeks.

It is clear that both types of attachment are equally powerful and effective. It is probably true that attachment grows more easily after early intimate contact between mother and baby. However, if there is a delay in establishing contact — for example, if the woman has a caesarean birth or if the baby is sick — normal attachment still takes place.

The Leboyer method of delivery, which advocates dim lighting and quietness at the birth, and immediate bathing of the baby in warm water, attempts to optimise the bonding process and to diminish as much as possible the 'psychological trauma' of birth to the baby. Most doctors agree that relaxation, comfort and lack of fear in the woman make her more receptive to her baby after delivery and also that quietness and calm in the environment are good for the baby and the bonding process. There is, however, no real evidence that bathing improves this situation or that other changes help. Indeed, there are very real dangers in exposing a wet baby for even a short time to the usual temperatures of an air-conditioned delivery room; these may be comfortable for adults but could chill a baby.

Some babies need help to start breathing
▼▼▼

There are two types of bonding between mother and baby
▼▼▼

It is certainly easy to believe that normal birth is traumatic to the baby: the pressure of the birth canal; the sudden transition from a soft marine-like world into bright lights and noise; and of course, the response to it all — the baby crying. However, there is no concrete evidence to support these theories and one must remember that the process of reproduction is extremely efficient, that babies are designed to be delivered and that at this time of life they are at their most resilient. Certainly conditions should be as good as possible at birth and any that are potentially dangerous or whose value is dubious should not be introduced.

*Not all skin
stretches
easily.*

▼▼▼

PERINEAL TEARS

Although the vaginal canal is capable of quite marked distension as the baby's head descends and injuries to it are rare in normal labour, this is not true of the opening of the vagina. Here the skin covering is quite thin and tends to tear easily if it is not allowed to stretch slowly as the head emerges. This problem is greatest with the first baby and naturally depends on the size of the baby and the size of the opening. Women over 35 having their first baby may have more fibrous tissue than the flexible elastic tissue of younger women. Bearing down in a totally uncontrolled way almost always produces a tear.

Tears tend to be irregular and usually extend backwards into the perineum, towards the anus. They may, however, be at the sides or the front of the vaginal opening and here may cause weakening of the

*Episiotomies
and tears are
uncomfortable
but they may
be necessary.*

▼▼▼

supporting tissues of the bladder, leading to a condition of urinary incontinence.

Such a condition, where urine escapes from the bladder on coughing, sneezing or laughing, is not uncommon for a few days after delivery, and is known as stress incontinence. It usually improves with regular exercising of the perineal muscles and rarely lasts more than one or two weeks.

EPISIOTOMY

When it is obvious that the skin of the vaginal opening is about to split uncontrollably, it is better if the doctor performs a clean cut with scissors rather than allow an uncontrolled tear or a series of tears to occur. This cut is called an episiotomy and is performed after injecting local anaesthetic to deaden the nerves. The cut begins in the middle of the back wall of the vaginal opening and is angled to one or other side to prevent any damage to the anus.

An episiotomy may be necessary in most cases of 'posterior' deliveries, in breech deliveries and in many cases of forceps delivery. When a perineal tear looks to be well controlled with the emergence of the baby's head, an episiotomy would not be required.

The advantages of an episiotomy over an uncontrolled tear are many. Apart from the better healing of a clean cut rather than a ragged tear, timely episiotomy can prevent widespread damage to the supporting tissues in the pelvic floor.

Naturally, the size of the incision depends on the circumstances and is never bigger than absolutely necessary. The episiotomy is repaired painlessly after the delivery of the placenta. An absorbable suture material is usually used, which does not have to be removed.

CAUSES OF A LONG SECOND STAGE OF LABOUR

Just as poor uterine contractions, a faulty position of the baby or a tight fit between the baby and the pelvis can cause delays in the first stage of labour, so too can they delay the second stage.

However, the delay now becomes more serious and corrective treatment more urgent. With the cervix fully dilated and the baby's head jammed deep in the pelvis, the upper uterine segment continues to retract with the usually powerful second stage contractions. As the placenta is attached to the upper segment, each contraction may interfere more with the oxygen supply to the fetus. The risk of fetal distress increases the longer the second stage lasts. Also, the continued effort of bearing down can exhaust the woman, so it often becomes necessary to assist the delivery.

A very common problem is failure of the baby's head to rotate into the occipito-anterior position. When this is the cause of the delay it is usual to rotate the head by a hand in the vagina, ventouse suction cup or special forceps. This can be done under local anaesthesia, a pudendal block, but an epidural block is usually preferred because of greater effectiveness.

In a few cases the head rotates into a completely posterior position and then descends further into the

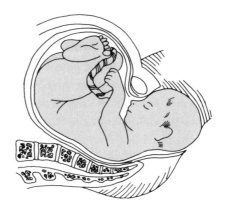

Delivery as a persistent 'posterior'

pelvis. This is known as a persistent occipito-posterior; some women deliver all their babies in this position. The baby sometimes has to be helped out with forceps or ventouse suction cup.

Occasionally the head assumes such an abnormal position that delivery is impossible and a caesarean section must be performed.

FORCEPS DELIVERY

The invention of obstetric forceps is credited to the Chamberlen family, a father and two sons, who first used them for delivery in England around 1600. One of them was even put into prison in 1612 for doing so, but was released after the intervention of the Queen and the Archbishop of Canterbury. The secret remained in the family for over 100 years and in fact the family line ended in 1728, but by then the invention had been sold. Over the next 200 years, modifications and improvements have finally produced the instruments in use today.

The indication for forceps delivery can be either maternal or fetal. Exhaustion and loss of emotional control in the mother can reach an extreme degree after a long,

There are many reasons for forceps delivery
▼▼▼

tiring labour and she may be unable to provide the extra effort to push the baby out. The forceps blades, lightly applied to the sides of the baby's head, are used to draw the head downwards through the vagina and over the perineum while the mother assists by bearing down. The forceps simply apply traction to the rigid bones of the face and do not exert pressure on the soft, flexible bones of the upper part of the head.

The main fetal indication is fetal distress as shown by irregularities in the heart action, particularly slowing heart-beat, and by the passage of meconium by the baby. The application of forceps to the head may seem to some to be adding to the baby's distress, but in fact it can cope with a reduced oxygen supply only for a limited time, and a fairly speedy delivery can be lifesaving. For the same reason an episiotomy in these cases is usually essential to reduce any excessive pressure on the baby's head.

Many women who have an epidural block need a forceps delivery as they lose the urge to bear down and forceps must be used simply to 'lift out' the baby's head.

In pre-term labour, despite the baby being comparatively small, forceps are sometimes used to provide a protective cage for the baby's head to protect its very soft skull bones from undue pressure during delivery. For a similar reason they are usually applied to the head in a breech delivery, not so much to speed up the birth but to slow down the otherwise sudden decompression of the head as it emerges. The forceps delivery of the head also reduces any risk to the baby's neck or shoulder nerves.

When the baby is a breech, different methods are needed

▼▼▼

For a simple lift-out forceps delivery it is often enough for the woman to be lying on her back with her knees well up. However, when it is necessary to rotate the baby and then deliver it by forceps it is usual for the woman's legs to be bent and elevated by the use of metal poles at the end of the bed, known as stirrups. Such a position (the lithotomy position) is not very elegant or comfortable. It does, however, provide the doctor with the best position for delivering the baby as safely as possible.

BREECH LABOUR AND DELIVERY

If the baby is coming bottom first it is called a breech presentation. Women whose pelvis is not very large or whose baby is larger than average are often delivered by caesarean section if the baby is a breech as there might be too many risks to the baby in a vaginal delivery. However, if there is enough room in the pelvis for a breech delivery, it is a relatively straightforward process with the necessity of careful manipulation of the baby's body and head.

Stirrups and an anaesthetic, either a pudendal or epidural block, are used and usually forceps to the head to control the delivery as the head in a breech delivery does not have time to mould (see page 110). An episiotomy is often performed.

TWIN LABOUR

Labour with twins is often quite normal particularly if both twins are presenting by the head. After the first twin is born, the second one usually follows within a matter of minutes as the cervix is already open. The doctor checks to make sure the second twin is in the right position and then probably ruptures the second bag of waters. Within five to 10 minutes the mother once again feels like bearing down and quickly pushes the second twin out.

If the position of the second twin is unusual, for example a posterior or breech, it will be necessary for the doctor to assist and proceed with the delivery in the usual way. Because of this uncertainty about the position of the second twin, it is usual to have an anaesthetist in the delivery room should an anaesthetic be needed quickly to relax the uterus, allowing intra-uterine manipulation.

THIRD STAGE: DELIVERY *of the* PLACENTA *and* MEMBRANES

After the birth of the baby, uterine contractions cease for between five and 30 minutes. Once they return, the contractions of the upper part of the uterus, where the placenta is usually attached, separate the placenta from the uterine wall by tearing through the loose tissue connecting them. A small amount of bleeding occurs (between 30 and 100 ml is usual) until the uterus forces the placenta through the relaxed cervix into the vagina. The empty uterus then closes tightly, compresses the blood vessels passing through the uterine wall, and bleeding ceases. The

whole process may take from 10 to 20 minutes.

Following the birth of the baby the uterus can be felt in the woman's abdomen as a soft round lump reaching up to the umbilicus. As it contracts and the placenta separates, the uterus becomes harder and rises above the umbilicus and the cord can be seen to lengthen by 5 to 10 cm.

The placenta can then be delivered by the woman bearing down or can be gently drawn out of the vagina by pulling on the cord, while the midwife supports the uterus with the other hand on the lower abdomen. In many parts of the world the woman squats and the placenta falls out. The membranes, which are attached to the placenta, are carefully withdrawn to avoid tearing them and leaving behind pieces which might cause infection. The placenta is always carefully inspected to make sure that it is complete and that no portion has been left in the uterus.

The main problem in the third stage of labour has always been excessive bleeding due to the failure of the uterus to satisfactorily separate and expel the placenta. However, for many years now it has been customary to inject a drug that will make the uterus contract and minimise bleeding. The drug usually given is a synthetic version (syntometrine) of the naturally occurring pituitary hormone oxytocin (uterine muscle contractor). It is injected into the woman's thigh muscle when the baby's shoulders are delivered. It produces strong contractions which cause the placenta to separate and be delivered within about three minutes (soon after the cord has been clamped and cut).

The placenta is delivered very soon after the baby
▼▼▼

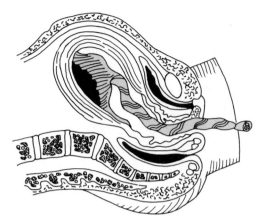

*Third stage of labour
Placenta separating*

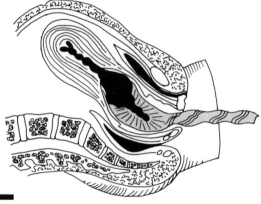

*Third stage of labour
Placenta separated*

---

*Some
problems
can be
anticipated.*

▼▼▼

Following the delivery of the placenta and membranes, any blood clots present in the uterus can be expressed by the midwife applying gentle pressure to the uterus.

Once the uterus is empty it remains contracted and this prevents any further significant bleeding.

Now is the time for a warm, relaxing, all-over wash, a general tidy of face and hair, a dry bed and a clean night dress. The next hour or two is for mother, father and baby to be together, to re-live the events of the day and happily plan for the future. The baby usually falls asleep after the initial sucking at the breast.

PREVENTION OF BLEEDING

Problems occurring during this third stage of labour may result in excessive bleeding which if not managed adequately can of course be dangerous. However, the effect of the oxytocic injection is to decrease the amount of blood lost during this stage of labour by up to 50 per cent.

Excessive bleeding can often be anticipated. It is most likely to occur after long labours, or when the uterus has been overstretched, as in the case of twins. A woman having her sixth or subsequent baby is also more likely to bleed heavily because increased fibrous tissue in the uterus can interfere with contractions. Also, in a case of placenta praevia, bleeding after delivery can be a problem as the placenta is attached to the lower part of the uterus, which does not contract.

In instances where the risk of bleeding is increased, special precautions are taken and in many cases blood will be crossmatched in advance in case it should be required urgently for transfusion.

CAUSES OF BLEEDING

Excessive bleeding after delivery of the baby is almost always associated with either failure of the placenta to separate properly, inadequate contraction of the uterus, or damage to the birth canal.

TREATMENT OF BLEEDING

If bleeding occurs and the placenta has not been delivered, then the top of the uterus is gently rubbed to try and stimulate a contraction to separate the placenta. Should this still not occur, further oxytocin is injected into a vein or into the thigh muscles, and the doctor will remove the placenta manually by inserting a hand into the uterus. If an epidural has been used during the labour no more anaesthetic is required but, if not, a general anaesthetic is necessary, although occasionally the nitrous oxide mask may be sufficient.

With the uterus completely empty, it can contract efficiently and bleeding usually stops promptly.

If bleeding continues after the placenta is delivered in the usual manner, it may be that the uterus, exhausted by its efforts during labour, is tending to relax.

The uterus will be felt through the abdominal wall and, if it is not firmly contracted, it will be rubbed to encourage this to occur. If this does not work, an intravenous drip containing oxytocic synctocinon may be commenced, and the bladder, if full, emptied by catheterisation, as a full bladder tends to encourage the uterus to relax.

Should the uterus now be firmly contracted but the bleeding persist, another source should be considered and this is most likely to be a laceration of the cervix or vagina. The lithotomy position (legs up in stirrups) is necessary to examine these areas and stitches are inserted to control the bleeding. Local anaesthetic is usually required for this procedure.

If in spite of all these measures the bleeding persists, a vaginal examination in the operating theatre under general, spinal or epidural anaesthetic may be required. The most likely cause is a piece of the placenta still stuck to the inside of the uterus.

During and after these procedures regular checks are made on the pulse rate and blood pressure and, if necessary, a blood transfusion may be given.

Problem bleeding occurs in about 15 per cent of women to a minor degree. A further 5 per cent lose more than 500 ml of blood and it is these women who are in potential danger and require quick appropriate treatment, which is available only in a hospital, if serious consequences are to be avoided. Blood transfusion is often necessary and in the presence of heavy or persistent bleeding, the sooner it is given, the better.

Blood is obtained from very carefully screened donors at the Red Cross Blood Transfusion Service, the screening of such donors being carried out by nurses. Following the screening the donor signs a statutory document and is liable for prosecution if any false statements have been given.

The blood is tested for a number of conditions, namely syphilis, HIV, and hepatitis B and C. The HIV testing procedure is very accurate in detecting infected blood.

In some cases sudden bleeding occurs hours, days or even some weeks after delivery. It is usually caused by a small fragment of placenta remaining in the uterus and finally separating. Often this bleeding can be controlled by an oxytocic and the placental tissue comes away naturally. If it persists, a general anaesthetic will be given and gentle curettage of the uterus performed if an ultrasound examination shows retained placental tissue.

Some placentas don't separate normally
▼▼▼

Not every uterus contracts properly
▼▼▼

Blood transfusion may be necessary
▼▼▼

CHAPTER 11

ANOTHER WAY TO HAVE A BABY

Caesarean Birth

Caesarean section is the delivery of the baby from the uterus through an abdominal incision. The origin of the operation has no association with Julius Caesar for it was performed hundreds of years before his time in the hopes of extracting live children from women who died in childbirth. The law governing this procedure was known as Lex Regia. It was later changed to Lex Caesaria and this is usually considered to be the source of the modern name.

Until about 1940 the thick upper part of the uterus was opened, but because of the risks of haemorrhage and infection associated with this, the operation of lower segment caesarean section has been adopted almost

A caesarean birth should not be feared

▼▼▼

universally. Despite this, there are still occasional indications for the older, 'classical' operation to be performed.

Forty years ago a baby was delivered by caesarean section only as a last, desperate resort. Today the procedure has become so safe that it has been accepted as the preferred method of delivery in many cases where the mother or baby are at risk. For delivery of a very pre-term baby, particularly when it is a breech presentation, the baby's chance of survival is statistically much better with a caesarean than with a vaginal birth. Nowadays the operation is used readily as a solution to many obstetric problems where previously vaginal delivery would have been performed.

The reasons for this change in management, particularly in the last two decades, have been the outstanding discoveries of the antibiotics and great improvements in anaesthetic techniques which have made the operation such a safe alternative to a difficult or dangerous vaginal delivery. The modern lower segment operation performed under ideal conditions, with the availability of blood transfusion and skilled medical care for the baby, bears no resemblance to the dangerous emergency operation of the first half of this century.

As mentioned in Chapter 8: *When should we go to the hospital?*, the decision to deliver the baby by a caesarean operation is sometimes made before labour begins and the procedure is then called an elective caesarean section. The common indications for this are:

1   A major degree of disproportion, where even a trial of labour is not justified, as it is known that the baby will not fit through the mother's pelvis;

2   Previous caesarean birth where the reasons for the first operation are still present, particularly disproportion;

3   Breech presentation, particularly in the first pregnancy if the maternal pelvis is smaller than average;

4   Placenta praevia, where the placenta lies in front of the baby and the onset of labour would lead to severe bleeding;

5   Some cases of severe hypertension;

6   Occasionally when the position of the baby in the uterus is totally unfavourable or when tumours such as fibroids prevent the head from entering the pelvis.

When problems arise during labour it may be necessary to perform an emergency caesarean operation. The usual causes are:

1   Fetal distress in the first stage of labour as indicated by changes in the baby's heart rate. If allowed to continue for too long, the resulting lack of oxygen could cause brain damage and ultimately death of the baby;

2   Bleeding from a placenta praevia or an accidental haemorrhage in the first stage of labour;

3   Obstructed labour due to disproportion which can only be adequately diagnosed during labour.

Some of the indications for caesarean birth can be recognised or strongly suspected during the pregnancy and wherever possible these women are admitted to a hospital with the best possible facilities for the operation and the subsequent care of the baby.

Even though it is so commonplace, most women find the prospect of a caesarean birth upsetting and alarming. As it is an abdominal operation, it has to be performed in an operating theatre, which is an area that is unfamiliar to most women and likely to arouse considerable anxiety. To make matters worse, no preliminary sedation is given before she is taken off to the theatre on a trolley, because any premedication might tend to make the baby sleepy.

Elective operations account for about half of all caesarean births

▼▼▼

The scar need not be ugly
▼▼▼

Bonding can be delayed
▼▼▼

Seeing the baby at birth can be very satisfying
▼▼▼

Generally, there is a choice between going to sleep under a general anaesthetic, or staying awake and having the operation under epidural analgesia. Most women, nowadays, choose to have their baby under an epidural block. If she chooses to go to sleep, she is usually not given any anaesthetic until the moment before the operation. This is to reduce the effect of the anaesthetic on the baby. The woman is lifted from the trolley onto the theatre table and asked to lie there breathing oxygen through a face mask for several minutes. After a catheter has been inserted to keep the bladder empty, her abdomen is painted with a cold antiseptic solution and sterile drapes are spread about her. Finally there is a quick intravenous injection and instant sleep until she wakes up in the recovery room about an hour later and is told the happy news.

A caesarean birth rarely takes longer than one hour and in many cases is completed in half that time. Nowadays the incision is usually made across the lower abdomen near the top of the pubic hair line and the scar of the operation is quite inconspicuous. This is popularly known as the 'bikini cut'. The incision is deepened to extend through the muscular wall of the abdomen to expose the lower half of the uterus. This is opened across the thin lower segment and the baby delivered through the incision. The placenta follows quickly and the rest of the operating time is spent in carefully sewing up the various layers.

When a general anaesthetic is given, there may be some delay in the establishment of breastfeeding and an inevitable interference in the bonding process between mother and baby. Every effort is made to minimise this, although there is no evidence of adverse long-term effects on the mother's relationship with the baby. The father is the first of the two parents to see the baby as it leaves the theatre and usually accompanies it to the nursery for the first examination and early observations. He is usually back in plenty of time to greet his partner as she awakens from the anaesthetic.

Many women find this way of having their baby a great disappointment For them it is more satisfying if they can be awake when the baby is delivered and they can see and touch it immediately. For this reason approximately 90 per cent of women ask for an epidural anaesthetic for their caesarean birth, with their partners present in the operating room to share this experience.

As far as the baby's well-being is concerned, there is very little to choose between the two forms of anaesthetic. There are some situations when the extra time required for an epidural may not be permissible because of a need for great urgency, particularly when there is fetal distress.

If an epidural has been decided on, it may be given in a small anaesthetic room adjacent to the theatre, and once it is fully effective the woman is taken into the theatre. By that time she will have become fairly numb up to the lower part of her chest, and will be asked to breathe oxygen from a plastic mask until the baby is born. A screen across the chest prevents her from seeing the operation, but she will be aware of some sensations of pressure and a little discomfort at some stages of the operation. The baby is born within about 10 minutes from the start of the operation and will be handed across for the first cuddle within another minute or two. Some mothers attempt to put the baby to the breast at this stage but the baby is usually too surprised at being born to take advantage of it. The paediatrician will soon whisk the baby away to the nursery where a thorough check is performed before the baby is left to rest for a few hours in a warm humidicrib. Mother can then have a doze for the next half hour while all the stitching up is done.

A caesarean birth under epidural analgesia can be quite an ordeal for a woman suffering anxiety, and no one should be persuaded to do this against her will. There may be some discomfort, and occasionally nausea is troublesome, but nearly all the women who have a caesarean birth with an epidural say they would choose it again, should a subsequent caesarean birth be necessary.

It is important for parents to realise that not all births are simple and uncomplicated. Some babies must be helped into this world, either by forceps or by caesarean birth or we would very quickly return to the bad old days of a high level of fetal mortality that previous generations experienced.

All too often, women who have had to have a caesarean delivery experience feelings of failure, disappointment and frustration. This is particularly so after an emergency operation where there may have been little time to accept and adjust to the changing situation. It is natural for every couple to have expectations of 'normality' and therefore to see any altered situation as 'abnormal'. However, the birth of every healthy baby is a success story, no matter how that birth is achieved, and there should be no grades of success in parents' minds. Regrets, recriminations and self-blame should play no part in the feelings of either parent over the birth process.

The success of childbirth is centred in the healthy baby, not in the performance of either parent.

A caesarean birth should not produce feelings of failure

▼▼▼

CHAPTER 12

IS MY BABY NORMAL?

The Newborn Infant

After nine months of usually deep but unexpressed anxiety, it is not surprising that the parents' first concern, following the delivery, is with baby's health and normality. Quite often the baby's appearance is not reassuring. The baby may be covered with blood (this is the mother's and is a natural consequence of delivery) or with vernix caseosa, the white fatty substance that is secreted by the fetal skin. There may be some bruises, the eyes may be bloodshot, and, most obvious, the head may be elongated or lopsided from the passage down the birth canal. All of these are effects of delivery; they disappear within a short time.

Apart from such transient phenomena the vast majority of babies are perfectly formed, yet it is sensible for every baby to have a full examination by an expert to check that all is well.

Baby's appearance may not be reassuring
▼▼▼

The first examination
▼▼▼

A second, more detailed check
▼▼▼

EXAMINATION *of the* NEWBORN

As soon as possible after delivery, every baby is examined briefly to check that adaptation to life outside the womb is satisfactory: that the lungs are working well, that the circulation is in order and that delivery has not caused any harm. If there are any major malformations or illnesses they will be picked up at this time and special care can be initiated as soon as possible.

A more detailed examination is then performed on all babies, ideally a day or so after birth.

The paediatrician obtains an enormous amount of information merely by observing the infant. The baby is best examined midway between feeds when neither full of milk and lethargic nor hungry and active. The baby's posture is distinctive: he or she lies with both arms and legs bent, head on one side and trunk straight. Baby breathes quietly about 40 times a minute but may periodically pant and then stop breathing for short periods of time. Baby's colour is generally pink, though often the hands and feet may remain blue and cool for a period after delivery. Baby's skin is observed for bruises from delivery and for birthmarks, such as the very common 'stork bites' (red marks usually on the eyelids, bridge of the nose or the back of the head), or the less common 'strawberry marks'. The palms of the hands are checked to see that the creases on them are normal, and also the fingers for normal fingerprints, as these are helpful clues to underlying problems; for example, palm creases are different in children with Down's Syndrome and other chromosomal disorders.

Following such observations, the doctor systematically examines the baby in detail from head to toe. By examining the baby from top to bottom (then on to the legs) only a little of the infant need be exposed at a time and baby can be kept warm.

HEAD

The head circumference is measured and tabulated. The soft spot (fontanelle) is examined for size and tension. It is at the top of the head, is diamond-shaped and easily indented with the finger. Despite its apparent vulnerability, the membrane covering it is very tough and there is no danger of injuring it with normal handling. Parents may notice that it sometimes pulsates with the heartbeat and bulges when the baby cries or strains. It usually closes by the age of 18 months.

The hair is fine and silky. The whorls and the way in which it lies can sometimes provide clues to underlying problems.

The eyes are usually blue-grey and clear. They may occasionally squint especially when the baby is feeding. This squint should not be constant; if it is, it may need correction. The lens and retina behind it are examined with an ophthalmoscope.

The ears, nose and mouth are checked for normal formation and position.

CHEST

The heart is examined carefully with a stethoscope for murmurs or defects. Most murmurs picked up in the first days are quite harmless, and are due either to the circulation adapting to life outside the womb or to tiny holes in the wall between the two main pumping chambers of the heart. Both conditions correct themselves with time, though are best kept under observation.

Also, the lungs are examined with a stethoscope to make sure the breath sounds are clear and normal.

ABDOMEN

In feeling the abdomen it is normal to be able to touch the edge of the liver protruding under the ribs on the right side. Occasionally the spleen can also be felt under the left ribs. Deep pressing reveals the kidneys, and their size and position are noted.

There are defects in the baby's skull bones
▼▼▼

Heart murmurs are not always serious
▼▼▼

INDIVIDUAL RESPONSES

Just as the labour and the method of delivery vary considerably from woman to woman and are largely unpredictable, so the reactions and responses vary in the first week after delivery. To some extent these reactions depend on the woman's personality, whether she is optimistic or pessimistic, calm or agitated, obsessive or relaxed, and on the expectations that have been built up during the long months of pregnancy. These expectations extend not only to the woman's own performance but also to the baby and, needless to say, are often somewhat idealistic.

EXPECTATIONS AND REALITY

Having been transferred to the post-natal ward, the ideal mother immediately leaps out of bed unaided, and heads straight into the bathroom. She obligingly passes a large amount of urine with no effort or discomfort, and glides back gracefully to her room, looking immaculate. Using several pillows and arranging herself in a comfortable position on the bed she puts her baby to the breast. The child is hungry and alert, and produces polite burps when necessary. She changes the nappy and cleans the umbilical cord with casual expertise. During the cuddle that follows the baby drifts off to sleep, secure in the loving bond that is now established. Back in the cot,

the baby will lie contentedly for exactly four hours, before stirring again to repeat the feeding process. During this time our mother opens her congratulatory cards from well-wishers, arranges the flowers that have arrived in great quantity and, after a refreshing shower, reclines in a maternal pose on her bed. She is now ready at visiting time to greet her partner, relatives and friends, with a warm smile.

There may be women like this and certainly there are many who paint such a picture of their own performance, often years after the event, when time may have dimmed their memories of the true state of affairs.

However, labour itself involves mental concentration and physical effort and can be a very tiring experience, particularly as it comes after the last few weeks of pregnancy when tiredness, insomnia and various aches and pains can make life miserable. Frequently the labour has continued through the night causing loss of sleep, and even the normal amount of blood loss at delivery aggravates the tiredness.

Immediately after delivery the mental and physical reactions of each woman vary according to the differing levels and lengths of stress experienced. Often the teeth chatter and the whole body trembles for five to 10 minutes. Tears are as common as smiles, although they are usually tears of joy or relief rather than of distress.

Idealistic expectations
▼ ▼ ▼

Reality
▼ ▼ ▼

The umbilical cord is examined. It should have three vessels (two arteries and one vein) and be composed of a jelly-like substance with a fibrous membrane over it. There are many variations in the appearance of cords; some are thick and fleshy and others thin and without much jelly. The skin may join the cord in a cuff half an inch out from the abdominal wall or the cord may apparently disappear inside with a prominent gutter around it. All these variations are normal.

In some babies a swelling may develop in or alongside the stump of the cord over the first few weeks. This is known as an umbilical hernia. It is not a cause for concern or for surgery as it causes no trouble for the baby and will gradually shrink and ultimately disappear over months or, in rare cases, years.

At the junction of the abdomen and the thighs the pulses of the main arteries of the thighs (femoral pulses) are located with the fingertip. If they are normal, it excludes the possibility of there being congenital narrowing of the aorta. Hernias in the groin are searched for and the genitals examined carefully for any abnormalities. In male babies, both testes should be in the scrotum (though they may be high up) by term. If, however, the examiner has cold hands, the testes may not be felt in the scrotum as the cold may have caused them to retract up into the groin.

HIPS

The hip joints are always checked for stability and to elicit any clicks present (see page 144).

LEGS

Many newborn babies have bow-legs, especially in the main lower leg bone (tibia). This is normal and the legs straighten with age. The feet also often curve in markedly; this is due to the position they occupied in the womb and it also corrects itself with time, especially when the baby starts to walk. Occasionally, some toes or fingers are fused together along some of their length. This often runs in families. If the fusing is likely to cause problems in later life, it may be corrected by surgery.

BACK

The baby is also turned over to verify that the back is normally formed and straight, and any dimples or marks examined. The anus is checked to make sure it is open.

NERVOUS SYSTEM

During the examination the doctor observes and notes the overall muscle tone of the baby, as well as mood, movements, cry and responses. Testing the baby's sight can only be approximate at this stage but he or she can be made to respond to light and brightly coloured objects and will follow their movement. Hearing may be tested to a limited degree by a loud noise such as a clap of the hands, which should startle the baby. However, babies will ignore such stimuli if they are tired, recently fed, distracted, or if the test stimulus is repetitive.

When the baby does respond to loud noises or other minor shocks it is with the Moro (startle) reflex. Baby flings both arms outwards as if to grab at something, then moves them in an arc towards the centre, then back to the chest. At the same time baby opens eyes wide, looks unhappy and often starts to cry. This is one of the 'primitive' reflexes; others are the grasp reflex (tickle the palm and see baby grasp whatever is in it), and an early walking reflex. All these reflexes disappear over the first weeks and months and by their disappearance indicate normal development of the baby's nervous system.

It is worth mentioning here that the newborn is really a very responsive individual; a baby can certainly see clearly and hear sounds; can also recognise and differentiate between smells (in particular own mother's milk as distinct from another's); baby can taste; and can respond positively to touch. Most surprising is the fact that baby will attempt to imitate a facial expression shown him or her, for instance sticking out the tongue, even within a few days of birth. And, when quiet and alert, baby will often attempt to synchronise movements with the cadence of the parents' voices, 'dancing' to the rhythm of words.

THE FIRST FEW DAYS

Adapting from a largely dependent state inside the womb to a physiologically independent existence outside involves many profound changes in the various systems of the baby's body. Usually the transition is a remarkably smooth one and no assistance is required. Nevertheless an explanation of some of these adaptive changes may help to allay the anxieties that parents often develop as they observe their new baby over the first few days.

HEAD

Following delivery, a baby's head may be strangely shaped for any of three reasons:

1   Moulding. Babies' heads are designed to alter their shape so that they fit through the birth canal. This involves the skull bones overriding slightly and is called moulding. Usually the change in shape rights itself within a few days after delivery. It is especially obvious with a first baby.

Depending on the way the skull bones have moulded, you can see which way the baby was lying inside the uterus. Sometimes the top of the head is elongated and sometimes the back of the head.

It is interesting to see the round heads of babies born by caesarean section, who have not had to force their way down through the pelvis.

2   Caput. Occasionally the part of the head which led the way down the birth canal is swollen and waterlogged due to an accumulation of bruising and tissue fluid. It is like a small round lump on the head. This also has no ill effects and disappears over the first few days.

3   Cephalhaematoma. This is an often large, soft swelling under the scalp but outside the skull, and is a result of bleeding from the outer layer

of the skull bone itself, caused by the trauma during delivery. Simply, it is bruised bone. It usually only occurs in babies who have been delivered vaginally. It is not related to any injury to the brain and if left alone the blood will be absorbed, in most cases over a couple of weeks. In 10 to 20 per cent of cases, this soft swelling gradually turns to bone. The abnormal shape may take some time to disappear, but it will gradually diminish as the skull is completely remodelled, and the baby's head will be a completely normal shape by three to four years of age.

TEMPERATURE CONTROL

Babies get cold quickly
▼▼▼

During this time take great care not to expose the baby to cool temperatures without adequate insulating clothing, as baby is unable to keep warm by increasing activity as adults can. Room temperatures of about 20°C (about 68°F) with the baby adequately clothed are appropriate.

URINATION

Boys can aim straight
▼▼▼

Most babies pass urine in the first 24 hours. If this does not occur, a reason must be sought. The urinary stream should be fairly forceful (mothers of baby boys usually receive a drenching demonstration of this early on!). If the stream is merely a dribble at best, it should be pointed out to the paediatrician.

BOWEL ACTIVITY

Virtually any bowel action is all right
▼▼▼

The first stool a baby passes, which is usually within the first 24 hours, is of the thick, black sticky substance called meconium, which lined the bowel while the baby was in the uterus. It is sterile and odourless. The baby continues to pass this substance over the first few days, gradually changing to normal baby stools once feeding is established. However, there is often confusion about what may be considered a normal stool habit for a baby. Breast-fed infants almost never have either diarrhoea or constipation and normality ranges from a stool as infrequently as one every three weeks to as many as 15 a day. The colour may vary from bright yellow through to green and the consistency from fluid to paste. Occasionally the stool may contain solid particles ('seedy' stool) and this, too, is normal. In short, in a fully breastfed baby, accept whatever is produced whenever it is produced. If baby has a stool only infrequently he or she may appear upset for a few hours beforehand and may be seen to strain and appear uncomfortable. As long as the stool is not hard, this is a normal phenomenon.

Bottle-fed babies, however, may occasionally suffer from constipation after a few days. They strain and push and produce hard, dry stools. This may be remedied by adding more water and some maltogen to their feed. This extra sugar draws fluid into the stool and softens it. Babies should not be given laxatives except under medical advice.

UMBILICAL CORD

Once the cord has been cut, it starts to wither and dry up and eventually falls off of its own accord. Until this occurs, which is usually within

10 days although it can be as long as six weeks, regular cleansing with methylated spirit is advisable to reduce the risk of infection. Parents are instructed in cord care before leaving the hospital. Usually, cleaning the cord and the gutter around its base with a cotton bud soaked in methylated spirit at each nappy change is all that is necessary.

Many parents are rather nervous about pulling on the cord in order to reach this gutter effectively, but this is essential and gentle traction will do no harm. Occasionally the cord may leak a few drops of blood during the first few days but this is not dangerous. Once it has separated, a granuloma may form at the point of separation. This is a damp, shiny, pinkish knob of healing tissue which may continue to weep fluid for some time after the cord has gone. It is easily remedied by the local doctor or baby centre. Usually the application of copper sulphate to the granuloma will cause it to disappear rapidly.

JAUNDICE

Nearly all newborn babies get some jaundice in the first few days. It is quite normal and bears no relationship to the jaundice which occurs in older children and adults.

While in the womb, the baby was not breathing but was obtaining the oxygen needed from the mother's circulation via the placenta. As this system is not as efficient as obtaining oxygen direct from the air via the lungs, baby required more blood (or more accurately, more haemoglobin, the red substance in blood cells) to carry the same amount of oxygen for

his or her needs. In addition, as a fetus baby had a special type of haemoglobin better suited to placental respiration. On emerging from the womb and converting to air breathing, much of this haemoglobin is now unnecessary and is therefore broken down. One of the main products of this breakdown is a yellow substance called bilirubin which, when accumulated in the body in large amounts, stains the skin and whites of the eyes the characteristic jaundice colour. This accumulation reaches its peak between three and five days after birth and then fades as the liver 'catches up' with eliminating it from the body.

If the staining is very strong, blood tests are run to monitor the bilirubin level and possibly to check for some disorders which might make the level higher than normal. It is important to keep the amount of bilirubin in the blood within safe limits, and so, if it appears to be rising to a high level, phototherapy may be used to control it. Bilirubin molecules absorb light from the blue part of the light spectrum and this breaks them down making it easy for the body to excrete them. Nowadays, this phototherapy is done in the ward with the baby remaining next to mother. Feeding is continued as usual and mother is encouraged to look after the baby in the usual way with the addition of keeping an eye on baby's temperature while baby lies naked under the light. Usually a baby will need phototherapy for no more than two or three days.

The cord dries and drops off
▾▾▾

The baby is born with more blood than is needed
▾▾▾

Jaundiced babies are quite healthy
▾▾▾

CLICKY HIPS

This fairly common problem is discovered on clinical examination of the baby and is a frequent source of misunderstanding and worry. During the examination the baby is placed on his or her back and the legs are flexed at the hip joint and pushed backwards in an attempt to move the round head of the leg bone (femur) out of the pelvic socket. The legs are then splayed out sideways. During these movements the examiner may feel 'clicks' around the hip joint. The commonest cause of these is quite harmless. After delivery the ligaments around the baby's hip joint (and everywhere else for that matter) are rather lax. This is due to the action of high levels of maternal hormones and the condition improves rapidly in the first few weeks. The lax ligaments may cause a click and this requires no treatment.

There are, however, other clicks which are not so harmless. In some babies the socket part of the hip joint is too shallow to accommodate the head of the femur in a stable manner, and testing the hips in the manner described causes the head of the femur to dislocate out of the pelvic socket and a very distinct clunk is felt. This is called 'congenital dislocation of the hip'.

In order for the socket to develop to the correct depth it needs the head of the femur to press firmly against it. If it is dislocatable that means that this may not be able to occur. It is very important that these babies are treated in their first few months because during that time the bones are soft and can be moulded (in fact they are only made of cartilage in the first year).

The treatment consists of a harness which causes the baby's legs to be flexed at the hip and this causes the firm pressure on the socket to occur. The harness is quite comfortable to wear and the baby is easy to manage as the nappy area is easy to get at. Usually it is permissible to take the harness off every now and again to bath the baby, and usually within a few weeks the problem is resolving itself to a degree that the harness can be removed. Progress can be followed by ultrasound examination and after four months an X-ray can assess the depth of the socket exactly.

Certain groups of babies have a greater likelihood of having congenital dislocation of the hip and these babies should be very carefully assessed not only clinically but possibly also by ultrasound. These are:

1   Breech babies

2   Babies who had a reduced amount of amniotic fluid in the uterus

3   Babies who have other evidence of a cramped intrauterine environment such as turned in feet

4   Multiple births

5   Babies who have an abnormal hip examination after birth

6   Those with a family history of congenital dislocation

This condition is also more likely to occur in girls and in first born babies.

Unfortunately, having a normal clinical examination at birth does not completely exclude the possibility of a potentially abnormal hip joint and ongoing hip examinations are well worth having. For instance in the first

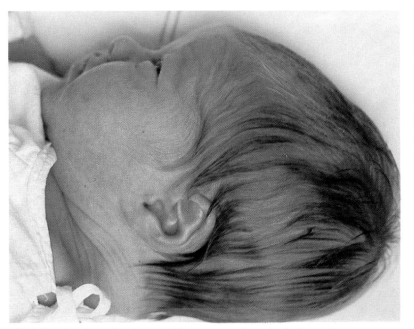

The baby's head may be elongated from passing down the birth canal.

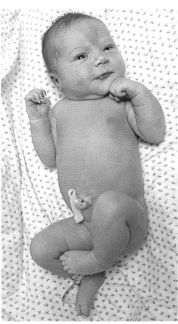

The characteristic posture of a newborn baby: arms and legs bent, head on one side, trunk straight.

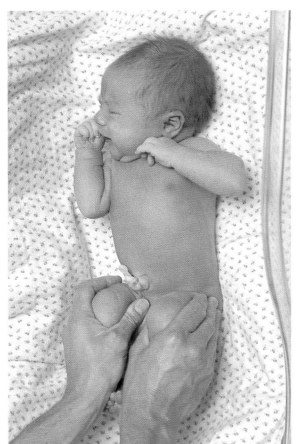

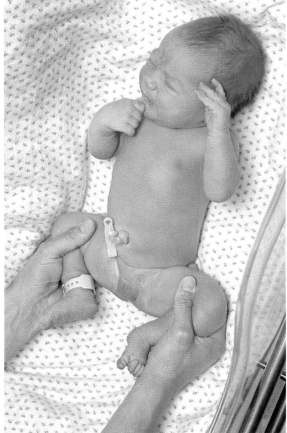

All new babies are tested for 'clicky' hips, which could be an indication of dislocated hips.

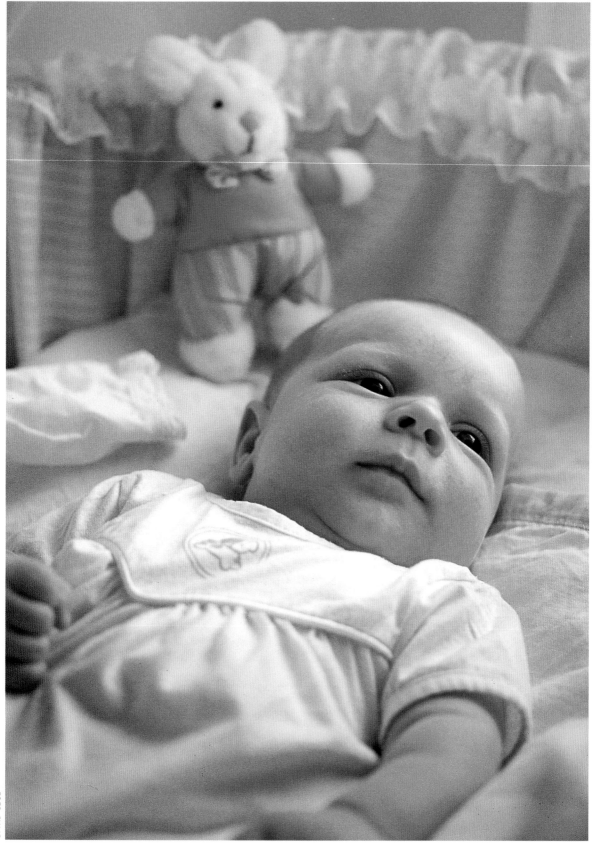

few months if the baby is lying on his or her back on the change table and the hips cannot be spread apart so that the knees touch the surface of the table, the baby should be re-examined by a paediatrician. Luckily these hidden hip problems are quite rare.

TOXIC ERYTHEMA

After one or two days, red spots with yellow or white centres may appear on the face and body. This is called toxic erythema. The cause of the rash is not fully known but seems to be related to contact of the skin with clothes, especially cotton. It is completely harmless and disappears after a few days.

FAT NECROSIS

Occasionally firm lumps may be discovered under the skin of the jaw or cheekbones on babies a few days old. Often they are associated with forceps deliveries. In addition, the skin overlying the lumps may appear red and inflamed. This is a harmless condition called fat necrosis. During delivery, fat cells under the skin may be ruptured by the pressure of the forceps blade or the mother's pelvic bone, and the fat which then leaks out sets up an inflammatory reaction around it. It resolves itself completely without treatment within a month.

SNUFFLES

A large number of babies develop snuffles and sneezes in the first few days and may keep this up for months. It may be severe enough to interfere with feeding or sleep but it is harmless. Only if the baby has trouble feeding should it be treated, and then only on medical advice. It usually starts within the first week of life and may be related to irritation of the mucous lining of the nose by either inefficiently swallowed milk or curdled gastric contents (see page 146). Occasionally, the mucus at the back of the throat may cause the baby to cough, especially at night. It usually clears up spontaneously at about three months of age.

MUCOUSY BABIES

Some babies vomit a lot of mucus gastric contents over the first few hours or days, and the first few times these may be mixed with old blood. This is simply blood which has been swallowed by the baby during delivery. The mucus, however, was probably not swallowed but produced by the lining of the baby's stomach in excessive quantities. The treatment is to pass a small tube down into the baby's stomach and wash out all the mucus and old blood. This may need to be repeated.

STICKY EYES

Quite commonly, a few days after birth the baby's eyes become sticky with mucus or pus. If the production of pus becomes very profuse, medical attention should be sought urgently. Usually, however, the amount is small and the only treatment required is bathing the eyes in sterile salt solution. If the condition continues despite saline bathing then treatment with antibiotic drops is often necessary. The eyes may also become

Red spots may appear
▼▼▼

More lumps
▼▼▼

Babies make funny noises
▼▼▼

Vomiting mucus
▼▼▼

watery. This often means the tear duct has become blocked with the debris of the infection. Massaging the nasal margin of the eye (tear sac) regularly and treating eye infections as they occur will clear most ducts in a few weeks. If the condition has not greatly improved by six months, syringing the duct clear by an eye doctor may be necessary.

VOMITING (POSSETTING)

In all of us there is a ring of muscle between the gullet and the stomach which acts as a valve preventing the stomach contents from re-entering the gullet when the stomach contracts. In newborn babies, this valve is not efficient and babies frequently bring up their milk especially when they burp. This is no cause for alarm but may become a nuisance. Sitting the baby up following his feed may decrease the vomiting. If it is severe, thickening the feeds of artificially fed babies may be necessary. However, this should only be done on medical advice.

BURPING

Babies do not really need to be burped. If a baby is cuddled upright after a feed and placed in the crib on the right side, he or she can bring up any swallowed air without help. If not, it will pass into the bowel, where it causes no discomfort or problem.

COLIC

Colic is extremely common and tends to recur in the evening. When it occurs the baby appears

uncomfortable and squirms, drawing the knees up and crying or screaming with apparent pain. This is often a tense baby with gurgling tummy who passes a lot of wind. Occasionally baby will be woken out of a deep sleep with a 'jump' and this will precede sometimes hours of crying. Typically, attacks are relieved by picking up and cuddling, feeding, or vigorous sucking on a dummy though occasionally nothing will calm the baby. The baby may calm down when being driven in a car, though will often resume screaming at traffic lights. This situation may create enormous family troubles with both parents frustrated, angry and often guilty about the anger they feel.

The old beliefs about colic are just myths and acting by them often makes matters worse. For example, babies who cry swallow air; hence crying babies are windy babies. The wind does not cause the crying — the crying causes the wind. Further, in nearly all cases there is nothing wrong with the baby's tummy. The baby does not need the milk formula changed, does not need posture feeding and has neither distension nor spasm in the gut. In nearly all cases the basic cause of the problem is tension, anxiety and frustration in the baby. Tension comes from the sudden change from the womb to the outside world, the inevitable increase in handling and exposure. Anxiety occurs because of the over-response of adults to crying.

Research on growing premature babies has shown that many babies are susceptible to overstimulation. Many things can arouse a baby — handling, joggling, rocking, the spoken voice and, especially, eye contact. There is a limit to the amount of stimulation a baby can cope with before being 'overloaded'. Unfortunately babies are unable to control the amount of imput when their limit is being reached and when this happens, the baby becomes tense and stressed. The baby may arch the back and make expulsive noises and generally look anxious. Also the baby will cry. Crying in humans is a normal mechanism for releasing stress and babies may use it for just that purpose. It does not mean that the baby is in pain or that something has to be 'done' to fix it. Indeed, it may be said that already too much has been done once the baby is overstimulated, especially as this leads to the baby being overhandled and made worse.

A parent's first action however should be to ensure that the baby is not hungry. Even if the baby fed only an hour ago, it is worthwhile checking this as a hungry baby will not be settled by other means.

Once fed, various techniques may be used to calm baby. It seems babies calm more easily when they are held in the fetal position (curling in) with the back rounded and the arms and legs contained. Holding the baby in this way within a sheet or blanket or by carrying baby in a sling is often helpful, otherwise deep warm baths may calm down an excited baby.

The only other important fact to remember is that no baby has ever been injured from crying, either physically or emotionally. Babies can, and occasionally do, cry for long periods without harming anyone but their parents.

PARONYCHIA

This is infection of the nailbed and is quite common. It appears around the sides of the nails as reddened swellings containing pus. It is worth getting medical advice and treatment if it is severe, but is usually treated just with local antiseptics.

BREASTS

Some newborn babies have enlarged breasts which may produce a little milky fluid in the first few days. This is due to maternal hormones acting on the baby. It is harmless to babies of either sex and the breasts will decrease in size in the first few weeks, or, maybe, months.

VAGINAL BLEEDING

Similarly, female babies may produce a mucous or bloody discharge from their vaginas during this time. This is also related to maternal hormones and is harmless.

HELP and ADVICE

The newborn baby has a tremendous adjustment to make in the first few days outside the womb. Most babies make the transition with great ease. Parents should certainly never hesitate to ask for help and advice.

Is baby hungry?
▼▼▼

Always ask for advice
▼▼▼

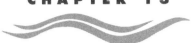

CHAPTER 13

WHAT ARE MY CHOICES?

Care of the Newborn

In the first few days after the baby is born, three important choices may have to be made.

Firstly, what sort of feeding for the baby: breast or bottle feeding? Whichever you choose, the midwifery staff will offer you support and advice.

The second choice relates to 'rooming-in': you may have to choose whether to have the baby with you 24 hours a day or only from morning till evening. This of course depends on the hospital's facilities; some hospitals are able to offer only partial rooming-in, whereas others may have facilities for total rooming-in.

The third choice is whether or not to circumcise a male baby.

There is a great deal of confusion about these choices and a great deal of conflicting advice will be offered. Most of this will ignore the basic desires of the mother.

Breast or bottle?
▼▼▼

In or out?
▼▼▼

On or off?
▼▼▼

FEEDING

The two main maternal activities directed towards the baby in the first few weeks are loving and feeding.

BREASTFEEDING

Nature has created the optimum food for newborns — the mother's breast milk.

Breast milk is unique in that it has great variability — offering the baby different tastes and textures as the milk matures.

At birth it is called colostrum — a sticky rich creamy coloured fluid that helps the baby's system adjust to new life. The first feeds give the baby not only concentrated protein **but** also immunoglobulins that protect the baby while his or her own immune system starts to develop.

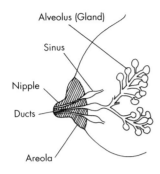

Alveolus (Gland)

Sinus

Nipple

Ducts

Areola

Correct position for sucking

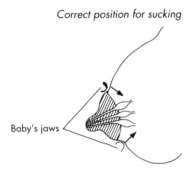

Baby's jaws

Colostrum also has a laxative effect which helps the baby pass meconium.

As the new milk 'comes in' and mixes with the colostrum during the hospital stay, the colour and texture of the milk begins to change. Mature milk has a bluish tinge to it and looks very much like skim milk. This is because breastmilk meets the baby's needs for fluids as well as food. Breastmilk is complete and meets the baby's nutritional requirements for at least the first four to six months. Nothing extra is needed.

Breastfeeding has advantages for the mother as well. Initially, as the baby feeds the mother's uterus is stimulated to contract to its pre-pregnant state, preventing excess bleeding. The fat stores laid down during the pregnancy to make breastmilk are utilised and weight is

gradually lost over the first six months. The hormones released during breastfeeding ensure good quality sleep and are important in the emotional bonding of the mother and infant. Long term there is some protection against ovarian and breast cancer.

Breastfeeding is convenient, is ready when baby asks to be fed and is cost effective as the immune protection baby receives ensures a healthy contented baby. The immunity conferred by breastfeeding continues on well into the second year of lactation.

There are no disadvantages to the baby from breastfeeding. The ones often cited are those perceived by parents to be disadvantages and can often be discussed and resolved with the midwife/lactation consultant during the pregnancy.

Starting breastfeeding

The production and release of breastmilk is the result of a fascinating chain of events. Once the placenta is delivered the hormones that begin milk production automatically increase in the mother's bloodstream causing the milk sacs to create milk. The frequency and vigour of the baby's sucking at the breast in these early days also stimulate this process.

The breast stores most of the milk in the milk sacs until the baby is feeding, then releases it into the ducts of the breast so it is available for the baby. This process is called the 'let-down' reflex. This reflex works automatically in the first few days, but gradually becomes triggered by the routine of feeding the baby and the response the mother has to the

Advantages
▼▼▼

There are no disadvantages
▼▼▼

baby. So in the first week when the mother hears the baby cry, she should arrange the pillows, change the baby, wash her hands, have a drink, put the baby to the breast and two to three minutes later the let-down will release the milk for that feed. Eventually she will fine tune this response and as she thinks about the baby her milk will be released.

For breastfeeding to be maintained the body needs both processes to happen: the stimulation by the baby of the breast to create the supply, and the release of the milk from the breast to create the room for more milk to be made.

Positioning of the baby at the breast

The two major discomforts of breastfeeding in the early days (tender nipples and overfull breasts) can be minimised by the correct positioning of the baby at the breast.

Mother: Comfortably seated, upright, back supported, or lying down next to the baby. Mother and baby's bodies should be close and relaxed — with no strain in their positions so the breast falls naturally into the baby's mouth. The shoulders can be covered to maintain privacy, but breasts should be as free of clothes as possible. There should be a glass of water handy.

Baby: Awake and alert, and unwrapped for skin to skin contact. Positioning hints:

Chest to chest
Turn baby's body so that it is facing yours. Support baby's body across your chest, level with your nipple. This is to prevent the baby's body weight dragging.

Wide open mouth
Wait for the baby to open wide — this enables baby to breastfeed not nipple feed.

Chin to breast
The baby needs more breast below the nipple in its mouth than above, so that the nipple points to (and sits in) the roof of the mouth. The tongue then curls up around the nipple. To achieve this the baby needs to come on the breast chin first. Your arm moves the baby's body towards the breast — the head is gently supported by your hand.

Deep rhythmical sucking
At the very start of the feed before you 'let-down' the milk, you will notice shallow sucking as the flow of milk is slow. Once you have 'let-down', the flow increases and this changes the baby into deep rhythmical sucking — indicating effective feeding.

Pain free
Some initial tenderness at the start of the feed is normal, due to the nipple being stretched. Once the baby's sucking rhythm changes this feeling should diminish. Pain is a warning sign — if you feel pain, take baby off the breast and start again. Checking the shape of your nipple once baby completes the feed can pick up early problems. The nipple should not look squashed or distorted.

How long should a breastfeed last?
Babies will often have long leisurely feeds, because food, security and love are all intertwined in the breastfeeding process. Sometimes the baby will have a brief snack and go back to sleep. The pattern of feeding in the first

week is very variable. They often don't develop a more predictable pattern until well into the second and third weeks.

Commonly babies do not feed frequently in the first 24–48 hours while they recover from birth and enjoy the rich satisfying colostrum. Just before the mature milk comes in they become more active at feeding — often seeming to feed all the time. Then once mother's breasts fill, become heavy (and maybe uncomfortable) the babies will start to space out their feeds again, though usually in a fairly erratic way.

There is a very good reason for this. The baby and the milk supply are trying to balance with each other. The baby's system is trying to adjust to the difference between colostrum and mature milk and the breasts are trying to produce the right amount of milk for the baby. Not too much or too little — but just right. This takes a little time.

The value of this time is that mother and baby are learning from each other. Mother is able to watch the changes in the baby's sucking pattern which tells her that the let-down is functioning. She can observe this pattern change from the 'suck/swallow/pause' — when there is a high milk flow to a 'suck/suck/suck/swallow/long pause' pattern — as the flow subsides. The feed finishes with lots of sucking and very little swallowing as the milk becomes thicker towards the end of the feed.

Allowing the baby to feed uninterrupted at the first breast before being offered the second breast ensures that baby gets a good balance of fluid and calories. It also means that as the mother observes the changes she learns her baby's individual pattern. This uninterrupted feed from the first breast also ensures that one breast is completely drained each feed — this makes her breasts more comfortable and synchronises her milk supply sooner to her baby's needs.

Should the baby fall asleep after the first breast and the unsuckled breast is uncomfortable the mother may need to express a little milk off until she feels more comfortable. This occasionally happens in the first week and the midwife will be able to offer other suggestions to keep her comfortable.

MINOR DISCOMFORTS WITH BREASTFEEDING

Tender nipples

Some initial tenderness is normal as the breast and nipple adjust to the baby's suckling. Damage to the skin integrity is caused either by the baby's incorrect positioning at the breast or by the inappropriate use of ointments and creams. Sometimes because mother and baby are learners skin damage occurs. The best treatment for this is to work with the midwife to find and correct the cause. In the meantime allowing the nipples to air dry for at least 10 minutes after the feed before replacing the bra, will encourage healing. The baby will leave a film of breastmilk on the nipples at the end of the feed — this not only is sterile but has a host of anti-infective properties in it.

Overfull breasts

When the milk 'comes in' the increase in milk volume and the needed

Feeding varies in the first week
▼▼▼

Let baby finish at one breast first
▼▼▼

increase in blood flow from which nutrients are drawn to make milk, can make breasts feel heavy, hot and uncomfortable. Allowing the baby to feed, uninterrupted at the first breast before being offered the second will assist at this time. The fullness is temporary — lasting about 24 hours, then the breasts gradually settle. Ice packs to reduce the volume of blood flow will often make mother more comfortable. Feeding baby at night is important for her comfort also. Fortunately baby takes 50 percent of his food overnight in the early weeks — so mother's and baby's needs can both be met. If mother is separated from her baby at this stage — the resolution of this overfullness may take longer to settle.

MULTIPLE BIRTHS

Once the skill of positioning both babies at the breast has been learnt — the joys of breastfeeding multiples can be enormous. With two breasts and two babies mother is rarely overfull as the breast adjusts quickly to the individual needs of each baby. She is in a unique position of overseeing the developing relationship between these new individuals. Contact with both the Multiple Birth Association (AMBA) and the Nursing Mothers Association of Australia (NMAA) can give her valuable practical advice.

BOTTLE FEEDING

When in hospital if formula feeding is desired, only one brand may be available. Baby formulas are very similar in order to standardise

formula preparation, eliminate mistakes in sterility and handling, and avoid unnecessary and unwarranted formula. It is a safe system and it works. However, at home use the formula you have most confidence in.

The technique of holding the baby, looking at the baby, relaxing and enjoying this contact is the same whether baby is receiving breast or bottle. The difference is the way mother feels. She may feel disappointed that she could not feed, or depressed and guilty that she did not want to feed or she may feel that the hospital staff are unnecessarily pressuring her to feed one way or the other. It is a free choice. The baby must be enjoyed as a person and how nutrition is received is not necessarily the prime factor in deciding baby's relationship with mother. Bottle feeding is certainly easy in hospital as the feeds come to the mother ready made (although at home preparing the formula may become something of a chore). Furthermore, the mother can see how much the baby gets, which some prefer.

BABY'S WEIGHT

In the uterus, the baby's body contains more water than it needs outside. This largely explains the loss of weight that virtually all babies experience during the first few days following delivery. Up to 10 per cent of the body weight may be lost during this period; there is no cause for worry.

As soon as feeding is established, the weight is rapidly regained, and this weight is real growth, not just water. Usually by the time of discharge from hospital the baby has regained the birth weight. Subsequent growth rates vary but on average it is about 30 g (1 oz) a day in the first few months of life.

BABY RELAXATION (A LOVING BOND)

Many parents are reluctant, some even frightened, to touch their baby. It is important that parents learn how to touch in a loving way. A deep, warm bath followed by a gentle massage is a therapeutic and enjoyable experience for the newborn. Both parents can participate equally and many fathers welcome the opportunity to be closely involved. A video of the Burleigh Relaxation Bath technique, developed at the Royal Hospital for Women, Paddington, is available from the Parent Education Centre.

ROOMING-IN

The postnatal period is the time when, in normal circumstances, mother and baby spend time together before going home. Bonding between mother and baby is established, and help is given with the day-to-day care of the baby. Postnatal care plays an important role in allaying any anxieties or problems.

GENERAL HOSPITAL WARDS

Today a common practice is 'rooming-in' whereby the baby is in the ward with the mother from early morning till early evening. The rooming-in regimen varies considerably from hospital to hospital. In some hospitals, all babies are returned to the ward nursery during visiting hours. Frequently there is a time set aside for partners only during the visiting period, allowing mother, father and baby and other children of the family to get together without other visitors.

MOTEL-TYPE ROOMS

An alternative to postnatal wards is motel-style accommodation. This type of accommodation is gradually being introduced in some hospitals and is becoming increasingly popular, as in the case of Herford House at the Royal Hospital for Women, Paddington, NSW.

Single rooms are provided and furnished as comfortable bedsitting rooms, so that the mother does not feel she is occupying a private hospital room. Not all mothers wish to spend their days alone, so a large lounge area is set aside for mothers to mix with each other and to entertain relatives or friends, creating a home-like atmosphere. Kitchen facilities and a dining area are also available as the majority of mothers prefer not to be made to feel as though they are ill after childbirth by being confined to bed for meals.

This type of care places a greater emphasis on the family unit as a whole and allows for greater bonding between mother and baby, who remain together on a 24 hour basis. It also differs greatly from the ward situation in that there are no set times for routines, so allowing each mother to establish her own routine for the care and feeding of her baby, enabling her to organise her daily activities in a way in which she can

Having the baby with you most of the time
▼▼▼

Having the baby with you all the time
▼▼▼

Family can become involved too

▼▼▼

You may need to be close to the nursery

▼▼▼

continue at home. As one ex-patient said: 'It was marvellous to go home and not have to change my routine.'

This type of postnatal care does not mean a drop in nursing standards and help is given to mother and baby by nursing staff, obstetrician, paediatrician, physiotherapists and others as required.

Whom does it suit?

This environment is suitable for any woman, whether it is her first baby or not. It is an ideal situation for the first-time mother, giving her the chance to get to know and understand her baby from an early age. It also suits the experienced mother as she feels free to care for her baby in her own way, free of rigid routines.

Those who have chosen motel-type accommodation for their post-natal care have enjoyed the relaxed atmosphere and feeling of freedom as well as the possibility of involving other members of the family. They appreciate freedom of choice in caring for their baby and the reassurance of knowing that the nursing staff are always there when needed. Not only does the mother benefit from this care, but also the father who too often tends to be forgotten. Here he is able to learn how to bath his baby and change nappies. And if there are other children in the family there is the opportunity for them to be involved with the new baby rather than feel rejected.

Other mothers who benefit from 'motelcare' are those who have given birth to pre-term or very sick babies. This often means a mother going home without her baby, who may remain in the nursery for several weeks. Just before the baby is ready to go home, she is able to return to the hospital and board for a few days, giving her the same opportunity to have the baby with her in order to gain confidence in handling her baby and to establish a suitable routine.

Whom does it not suit?

Motel-style accommodation does not suit anyone who does not wish to have her baby with her 24 hours a day. This may be a totally normal reaction in many and should not be frowned upon. Also, many women feel isolated in single room accommodation and prefer to share a ward with others.

In some circumstances a baby may require more intensive nursing in a special care nursery, so mother and baby are separated. Many mothers in this situation are better placed in a ward close to the nursery where often there are other mothers whose babies are in the nursery.

Mothers who are not well enough to care for their babies at first, for example those who have had a caesarean section, can move to the rooming-in area after several days and remain there till they return home.

WHICH TYPE OF CARE?

This depends on the mother. Some prefer not to have the baby with them all the time. Others prefer not to spend any time in a postnatal ward, but to be totally involved in the care of their baby. Many women prefer to spend the first few days in a post-natal ward and then change to motel-type accommodation.

CIRCUMCISION

There are few subjects in medicine so surrounded by myth and magic. This ritual operation is now falling more and more into disfavour.

Leaving out the Jewish and Muslim members of our community, less than 10 per cent of boys are circumcised today. Consequently boys do not need circumcision in order 'to be like all the others', although brothers probably do want to be the same in this area. The only really important question is whether or not it is needed medically. And the answer is emphatically 'No'.

Nevertheless parents are extensively pressured by their parents, relatives, friends and others to accept circumcision. It may be very hard to avoid these pressures. A few years ago there were some reports that the sexual partners of uncircumcised males had an increased incidence of cancer of the cervix. This has been found not to be the case. Similarly, there is no real evidence that circumcised men are better lovers.

Many parents are concerned that their son may need to be circumcised later in life. This is necessary only if the foreskin is over-handled and damaged when it is being cleaned, if it is forcibly retracted while it is still attached to the head of the penis or if recurrent infection occurs.

In only 5 per cent of newborns is the foreskin retractable and the other 95 per cent can be left alone for the foreskin to separate of its own accord from the head of the penis, which may take anything up to four years. If retraction is forced before then, scarring may occur and the result will be a narrow foreskin which is impossible to retract when the boy is older.

Recurrent infections behind the foreskin (balanitis), can develop for two reasons:
1   Inefficient hygiene. Naturally the little boy must be taught to wash behind his foreskin as soon as it is retractable.
2   Narrowing of the foreskin (phimosis). This makes the foreskin impossible to retract and leads to a lack of hygiene. It is usually caused by wrong management of the uncircumcised baby, by the forcible retraction of the foreskin before it has separated from the head of the penis.

Most paediatricians today do not recommend circumcision, but, rather, leaving the foreskin alone until the boy is three or four years old. Then he should be taught to wash behind it, and it will give him no trouble. For a baby it is an advantage to have a foreskin as it prevents his sensitive glans from being affected by nappy rash and avoids the possibility of a small ulcer developing at the opening of the urethra (meatal ulcer).

Keep in mind that it is an operation that can cause illness and, in exceptional circumstances, even death.

Some people would say that no child should be circumcised unless he personally asks for it!

Circumcision is not necessary
▼▼▼

Efficient hygiene minimises infection
▼▼▼

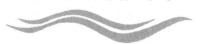

CHAPTER 14

WHEN CAN WE GO HOME?

Postnatal Care

One of the first questions asked by a woman with her newborn infant is 'When can we go home?' If all the support and caring systems were available at home there would be little need for postnatal stay in obstetric hospitals and the patient would be able to go home early.

In many countries there are efficient nursing and medical services which provide adequate postnatal care within the home, so women and babies leave hospital after 24 to 48 hours. In other countries hospital treatment is so expensive that cost dictates early discharge, while others have such an inadequate

Five days is the norm

▼▼▼

hospital system that there are just no beds available.

Traditionally Australian new mothers have stayed in hospital after delivery for about five days and our hospital system has been geared to this concept, although at times of rapid population growth this has had to be reduced to about three days. Whether the postnatal care is given in a hospital setting or at home, there is no argument about the need for care and for greatly reduced activity in the first three to four weeks. Early discharge programmes are available and should be discussed with the midwife or doctor.

EMOTIONAL REACTIONS

*One and one
make three*

▼▼▼

Each woman's experience in the first few days after delivery is unique to her. Also she will find that feelings differ from baby to baby, so she never repeats with her second child the emotions that went with the first. However, there are a few typical reactions and feelings for the new mother.

Once the baby has arrived, the woman's feelings are confused. Labour will have left her feeling tired but elated. The months of waiting are over, the baby is lying on her tummy and she has been told all is well. Should she cry, should she laugh? Probably a bit of both as she has just experienced that most wonderful of miracles, the birth of a healthy baby. A quick look at the father will show him also smiling with tears in his eyes but not just for baby, also for mother. Many a woman at that point thinks or asks, 'When can I do it again?' Many another thinks 'Never again.'

Then mother, father and baby are alone. Whatever the doctor or nurse has said, most parents want to satisfy themselves that all those fears about the baby were unfounded and check the baby carefully. Ten toes and fingers, two perfect arms and legs and a swollen little face. There is joy in discovering minute finger nails, shell-like ears and everything there but in miniature. Only then can mother and father give in to relief and rest.

*Doubt and
disappointment
is natural*

▼▼▼

By the time the baby has been cleaned up and the mother has rested she is ready for another look. Many women will have visualised what their baby would look like, what sex it would be and what disposition it would have. On the second look at the sleeping bundle in the basinette sometimes doubts start to creep in. Perhaps the baby is not everything the mother had imagined. Maybe a twinge of disappointment is felt and even out-and-out dislike for the child can well up. Is this little stranger all there is going to be after the long waiting months?

Inevitably, partner and grandparents, aunts and uncles come pouring in, gushing over the beautiful baby. How can one share with them the doubts and uncertainties? A newborn baby fortunately needs a lot of sleep so is not likely to cause too much rumpus and will tolerate fumbling efforts to change a nappy, uncertain handling of the tiny little body and the mysteries of feeding.

Many women experience this uncertainty in the first 24 hours. Another good sleep and they take another look: the baby really does have some cute little ways and perhaps does not look so bad after all. The relatives have picked out all the family features and in this way have incorporated baby into the family as one of them. If mother looks really hard she may well find that baby does have father's chin or her eyes. By around the third day the baby really is the most beautiful child that ever was. All these feelings are normal.

Women not having their first baby usually find they can get to know the new baby rather more quickly than the first time. They know the doubts are unfounded and the disappointment does not last. They know they are not perfect mothers and do not expect perfect babies.

In very rare cases, however, the feelings do not go away. The baby stays a stranger and the disappointment that the hoped for 'dream' baby did not eventuate, remains. Mother finds it hard to love the baby and can feel the child's crying, soiling of nappies and other behaviour is designed to upset her and make her life difficult. This is serious and must be mentioned to her doctor or hospital staff. Help is available for such a mother and taking advantage of it straightaway is likely to prevent any more serious problems occurring in the future.

TRYING TO MANAGE

For a new mother, handling her first baby can be a nerve-racking experience. Even the most competent woman can find her self-confidence and common sense desert her as she is confronted with this tiny, squealing, wriggling body. Women who have been used to succeeding at whatever they do, find this a disconcerting experience that can leave them frustrated and anxious. Feeding often presents even more problems. Just getting the nipple in the baby's mouth can be hard enough, but if baby will not suck, goes to sleep on the job or the nipples become cracked and sore, it is even worse.

A woman can become anxious, tense and exhausted with all of this. Relaxing and counting to 10 before trying will often help her draw on her own common sense and initiative. It helps to remember that she is smarter than the baby. Then by proceeding slowly and calmly, softly talking or even singing to baby, gradually everything will fall into place. Nursing staff have all sorts of handy hints but it is not wise to try them all

at once. It can be confusing if advice is contradictory, but if there are specific difficulties it is worth listening to the advice and trying it out. If it does not work, do not hesitate to reject it, as not everything works for everybody.

Many new mothers have never been in hospital before. They can be overwhelmed and it is easy for a woman to feel intimidated if she sees staff as super-efficient and knowledgeable. It is important that she overcome this; staff are there to look after her needs, not the other way around.

Inevitably as the mind and body relax after delivery, tiredness occurs and most new mothers appreciate a period of rest over the next few days. The feeling of fatigue gradually passes and the lack of sleep is made up slowly, mainly by short extra periods of sleep during the day. 'Quiet times' when visitors are not allowed and no nursing routines are performed are an important element of hospital and home care. There is a lot to be said for restricting visitors for the first few days to partner and immediate family, for a tired and over-stimulated mother often has problems with breastfeeding and infant care.

POSTNATAL BLUES

There are many theories about those tearful, depressed days that occur for many women somewhere between three and five days after delivery. The common feature of all these theories is that the feelings are normal and probably uncontrollable.

Is it any wonder that after the build-up to the delivery, the trauma and excitement of giving birth and

It is normal to be nervous at first
▼▼▼

Only take the advice that works for you
▼▼▼

Please, not too many visitors
▼▼▼

the happy but tiring and emotionally draining days that follow, it all becomes too much and the new mother reaches for a tissue? They are not tears of sadness or feelings of real depression, but more a feeling of being overwhelmed by all that has happened and the awareness of the responsibility for what is going to happen.

Suddenly there is a tiny, defenceless person dependent on her for every need for 24 hours of every day. It can seem a huge burden and fears of not knowing what the baby wants, of not having enough milk and of generally being unable to nurture the baby, arise. Also the baby does little to cheer her up. Once the milk begins to flow at about three days, baby may become very demanding from a breast which is still inexperienced and may be tender from either engorgement or sore nipples. This can increase the mother's feeling of inadequacy and depression. It is at this time that she needs most support from partner, medical and nursing staff, as it is easy for her to contemplate giving up breastfeeding because she sincerely believes it would be best for her baby.

Every woman wants to be a 'good' mother. This is an expectation that she not only has for herself but so does everyone else. They are confident she can do it, while she often feels totally inadequate to the task and quite isolated. These fears of being unable to cope with the future can be heightened if the woman's own experience of mothering was poor as she will be trying to do things differently from the way she has seen her own mother do them and yet does not have a good

model to copy. The woman's body is still undergoing a lot of changes as it returns to its pre-pregnant state and lactation is established. This is all likely to leave her feeling less than 100 per cent fit, physically and emotionally. About this time, despite all the flowers, cards and well wishes, the mixture of emotions can be overwhelming This can leave her feeling down and uncertain and sometimes guilty. Perhaps the best way to deal with all these feelings is to let the emotions flow. Crying is a good release for pent-up emotion and many women feel much better for a good weep.

These tearful feelings rarely last more than a day or two, and the fears of inadequacy disappear. As she gets into a routine with the baby, feeding becomes easier and as she feels stronger and less tired, the future begins to look manageable. The rosy glow has gone and she is starting to look forward in a more realistic way and, most importantly, is realising she will be able to manage.

CONFIDENCE

This aspect is best illustrated by the question 'What do I do when my baby cries?' The answer to this is that the baby is communcating to the mother about requirements that may be one of the following: hunger, loneliness (not common), discomfort (e.g. from a wet nappy), and so on. A systematic approach which may be difficult at first will be successful in the long run and after a short period, confidence and recognition of baby's call will be interpreted correctly by the new mother.

Feeling sad can be normal
▼▼▼

A good cry can help
▼▼▼

Do what you feel is right
▼▼▼

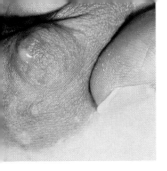

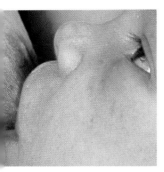

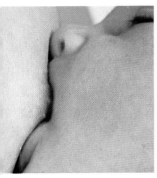

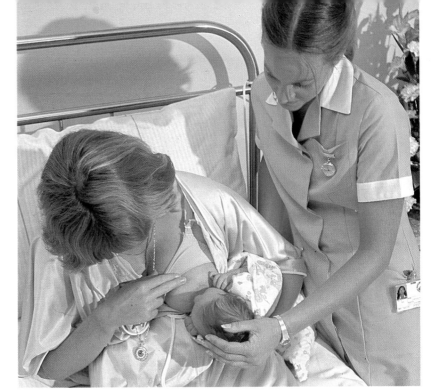

Above: For some mothers, under-arm feeding is more comfortable.

Left top: Mother offering the nipple as though it were a bottle teat.

Left middle: Baby sucking the nipple as though it were a bottle teat.

Left: Baby correctly 'attached' to the breast.

Below: Twins usually wake together, but sometimes one may have to be woken in order to feed them both at the same time.

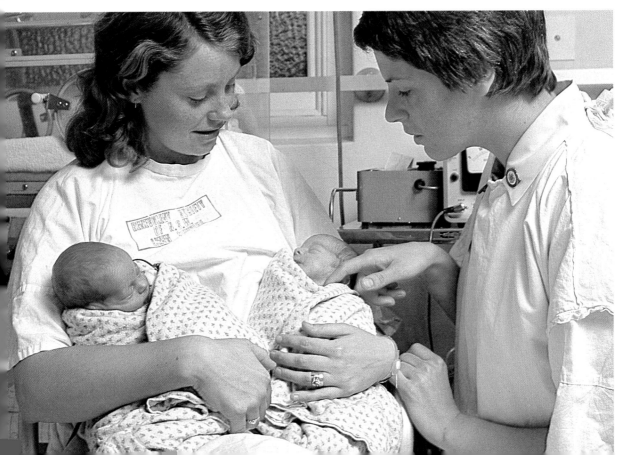

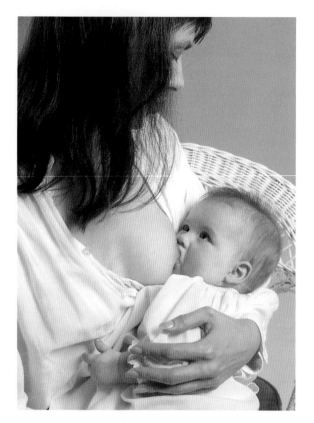

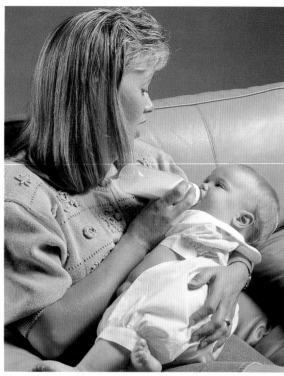

Relaxing and enjoying close contact with your baby are the same whether you breastfeed or bottle feed.

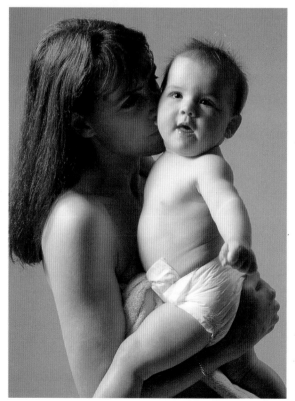

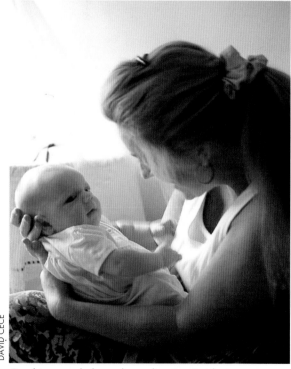

DAVID CECE

Touching your baby and spending time just loving are important in forming a close relationship.

WE GRATEFULLY ACKNOWLEDGE HJ HEINZ CO. AUST LTD FOR SUPPLYING PHOTOGRAPHS TOP LEFT AND RIGHT AND BOTTOM LEFT

OTHER CHILDREN

While a mother with her newborn infant is in hospital it is important that the feelings of her other children, especially if they are under four years of age, be considered. If they are not used to her being away from home and she has disappeared rather suddenly, it can be confusing and frightening even if they have been prepared. The commonest fear is that she will never come back.

It is important that children visit their mother in hospital as often as possible to see that she is still around and not far away. Nonetheless some children will show an angry response, and the longer the separation, the greater the anger. Typically they may refuse to recognise her, to talk to her or even smile at her in the first few visits. Then they may become clinging and object to others approaching, touching or talking to her. It may be difficult to take such children home after a hospital visit.

Despite this behaviour it is important that the child knows that mum is still around and continues to be interested. When it is impossible for the child to visit mother, phone contact at least is important for the child to be reassured that she still exists and cares for him or her.

These reactions seem to occur no matter who looks after the children and how happy they seem to be. The more the child understands the situation, the less likely the separation will produce any deep or problematic effect. This is why the younger children are more likely to be affected.

SHRINKING (INVOLUTION) *of* the UTERUS

In the first 10 days after delivery the uterus shrinks quite rapidly from the size of a grapefruit to that of an orange. Following delivery it weighs 800 g and in the next six to eight weeks it returns to its pre-pregnancy size and weight of 40 g. This dramatic change is accomplished by a continuous reduction in size of the giant muscle fibres produced during pregnancy.

The numerous large blood vessels in the pregnant uterus become blocked as the blood clots inside the vessels and fibrous tissue grows into the blood clot. As this fibrous tissue shrinks, the vessels are reduced to thin cords which ultimately disappear.

At the same time the thick lining of the uterus gradually strips off and finally returns to a normal, thin resting layer in about six weeks.

All of these changes cause a discharge from the uterus known as the lochial discharge. For the first few days it is red, mainly liquid blood with a few small clots. Later it will be brown and finally yellow when it is composed entirely of fragments of the lining of the uterus and tissue fluid squeezed from the contracting, involuting uterus. For the next few weeks some further bleeding may occur, often associated with extra activity but this should not be interpreted as a menstrual period. The lochia usually remains coloured for three to four weeks but it is not unusual for it to persist for twice as long.

The uterus loses weight
▼▼▼

Lochial discharge usually lasts for four weeks
▼▼▼

GENERAL CARE AFTER DELIVERY

In the absence of complications, most women get up to go to the toilet within six hours of delivery. As water is retained by the body during pregnancy, quite large volumes of urine may be passed in the first few days following delivery. On the other hand the bowels are normally sluggish, so the diet should contain adequate roughage with fresh fruit and fruit juices to prevent constipation. The congestion and stretching of the perineum in labour extends to the anus, and haemorrhoids often appear after delivery. These are usually external rather than internal and are caused by small veins under the skin breaking and causing painful swellings. They settle down spontaneously in a few days, but if not, ice packs and anaesthetic creams can be used for pain relief.

Within 12 hours of delivery, most women shower. The use of flexible shower hoses (perineal showers) has largely removed the need for nurses to swab the perineum even in the presence of stitches and greatly improves the comfort of the perineum.

As the discomfort of sore pelvic muscles and a bruised or lacerated perineum can make walking uncomfortable and lengthen the process of full recovery, activity is best restricted to these functions for the first few days and rest in bed still remains the best method of recovery, with a little mild exercise if comfortable. Also, in a standing position, the softened ligaments allow the heavy uterus to fall downwards into the pelvis. Any tendency for the uterus or the bladder to prolapse later in life may be increased by too rapid a return to activity and particularly by any heavy work.

The appetite is almost invariably good following delivery but care must be taken to continue with a nutritious diet if weight gain has been a problem during pregnancy. The chocolates supplied by well-wishers are much appreciated by visitors, nurses and doctors but should play very little part in the nursing mother's diet.

NUTRITION

Good nutrition is as important to the breastfeeding woman as it was during pregnancy. The needs for nutrients and energy are increased and, as the baby grows, it becomes necessary to eat more to satisfy the appetite and to maintain the increasing milk supply.

What to eat becomes more important than how much, and highly nutritious foods such as milk, meat, chicken, fish, cheese, eggs, cereals and bread are important items. Snacks between meals may be necessary, but at all times choose good foods. Fruit and fruit juices are important for their vitamin C content, and milk, water and fruit juices should be increased in response to thirst.

Many substances can be transmitted through the breast milk and may affect the infant. Some women find that certain foods such as prunes, stone fruits, chocolate, low-calorie drinks and spicy foods upset their babies. Others can eat anything, so a certain amount of trial and error is necessary.

Many easily available drugs such as aspirin, laxatives and sedatives can pass into the milk and medical advice

Go slowly
▼▼▼

You don't have to drink milk to produce milk
▼▼▼

should be sought in this regard. Cigarette smoking decreases milk production and the nicotine also passes into the milk, as does alcohol. A small amount of alcohol is not thought to be harmful, but it is certainly not beneficial.

When weight gain during pregnancy has been the average of 10 to 12 kg, this amount will usually be lost during the first three to four months of breastfeeding so that dieting is usually unnecessary. If this does not occur naturally, it may be necessary to commence a low kilojoule diet with an extra allowance for breastfeeding, say a 7100 kilojoule (1700 calories) diet as recommended by a dietitian.

For those who are not breastfeeding, much closer attention to diet is necessary, the aim being to return to the pre-pregnancy weight within six months.

POSTNATAL EXERCISES

The reasons for doing postnatal exercises are very practical. Every woman wants to regain or, better still, improve her pre-pregnancy fitness and health. She also wishes to gain good tone in all the muscles and ligaments affected by pregnancy and labour. She endeavours to re-establish good respiratory and circulatory function and assist involution of the uterus. Perhaps most of all she wishes her first few days after delivery to be as free as possible of any complications, so that she can enjoy her baby.

Early movement and sensibly graded exercises are of great assistance in making these wishes become a reality. As with prenatal

exercises, exercise does not have to be complicated to be effective and the same two rules apply: do not do anything that hurts and do not overdo it. Remember also that some muscles of the body, namely abdominal, back and pelvic floor muscles, have undergone great strain. But also be assured that this strain is capable of being endured by the muscles and that it is possible to restore them to normal function. Another maxim to keep in mind is that no one gets better lying still and despite the odd ache or pain (most frequently from stitches), every new mother is encouraged to begin some exercises on her first day after delivery.

This may merely consist of simple breathing and leg exercises, abdominal muscle contractions and continuation of the pelvic floor contractions.

Position for exercise is important. The most suitable position is to lie with a pillow under the head, not the shoulders, and on top of the bed clothes. This position allows good support for the back, little or no pressure on the pelvic floor, and puts the abdominal muscles into the best working position. Above all it is a position of comfort.

As exercise is upgraded, so positions may be altered — sitting and standing. However, no matter how simple the exercise may seem, no one should attempt raising one or both legs without the knees bent. This places incredible strain on the lower back and could do irreparable harm. Exercise should also be upgraded according to the woman's rate of recovery in every sense. Too much too quickly will have an adverse effect both physically and psychologically.

Exercise carefully after delivery but don't lie like a log

▼ ▼ ▼

POSTURE

Posture is still important, in all positions. Side lying with one leg bent well up, pillow cuddled into the abdomen just below the breast, will still be a favourite with lots of women. But now, with the bulk of the pregnant uterus gone, lying on the stomach is possible. This can be indulged in to the heart's content, with bonuses: the added pressure on the uterus helps to stimulate involution and the back gets some needed respite. Some women may prefer a small pillow under the hips when lying face down. This will prevent any hollowing of the lower back. Comfort will decide whether it is needed or not.

In reclining or sitting, care should be taken to ensure that the lower back is well supported on every occasion, particularly when feeding the baby. This should be a time of rest and relaxation as well as for fulfilling the needs of the baby.

Posture in standing is again the hardest to maintain. The first things to consider are the changes that have taken place in the body during and following birth. The main ones are loss of bulk and weight. As the abdomen is now much less stretched, the muscles respond more easily to exercises. Despite the absence of the baby inside the uterus, most women find that their abdomen continues to protrude, especially when standing. The same rules of posture apply as before. Stand tall with the weight evenly distributed over both feet, knees not pushed hard back, pelvis tilted upwards in front by holding the tummy muscles as firmly as possible,

back flat, chest relaxed forward slightly, shoulders relaxed, head at a normal angle, and above all, breathing easily. Using a wall as a support and then stepping away from it is an easy way to check posture. As the postnatal period progresses so the need to alter and re-check posture will be necessary.

SPECIAL PROBLEMS

EPISIOTOMY AND STITCHES

Whether the perineum has been torn at delivery and subsequently stitched or whether an episiotomy has been performed, the sensation will be the same. The perineum will be tender and painful for 24 hours if only skin or superficial tissue have been torn or cut. Discomfort for a longer period is due to the stitches repairing the torn or cut perineal muscle. This muscle contracts both consciously and unconsciously, every time the mother coughs, laughs, rolls over or stands on one leg, and so pulls against the repairing stitches. Sometimes a deep bruise affects the muscle, and this will cause pain for a few days until the bruise softens. Nowadays, the stitches are usually of a dissolveable material.. As they do not have to be removed they are not counted, something which older generations may have difficulty in understanding.

FORCEPS DELIVERY

Where this has been a simple lift-out forceps delivery, possibly associated with an epidural block, the sensation

Lying on the tummy can be heavenly

▼▼▼

and responses after delivery will be identical to a normal birth. Where there has been some difficulty in delivery, possibly with an episiotomy and some bruising of the vagina, there may be problems in passing urine. This will usually be solved by sitting up but occasionally the bladder becomes over-distended and a catheter will be inserted to drain the urine. Occasionally the catheter will need to remain for 12 to 24 hours with the urine draining into a plastic container.

CAESAREAN SECTION

When a caesarean birth has been necessary, the return to normal activity will be slower. The rate of immediate recovery depends on whether there has been a long period of labour before the operation or whether it has been performed prior to the onset of labour. Equally it will depend on whether a general anaesthetic or an epidural block has been used. With the former there are the usual post-anaesthetic problems of nausea, possibly vomiting, and often a sore throat due to the anaesthetic tube inserted through the mouth into the windpipe. With an epidural block there will be none of these but in both cases the operation itself leads to a very sore abdomen for 24 to 48 hours. Also the abdomen will be more distended, and colicky pains will occur for the first 48 hours until some wind is passed through the bowel. Thereafter the recovery is rapid.

Postnatal exercises need to be modified after a caesarean birth and the mother will usually be in hospital for a few extra days.

MULTIPLE PREGNANCY

Because of the large size of the placenta and the greatly distended uterus, there is likely to be more bleeding after twins or triplets are delivered. The involuting uterus is bigger and there is a greater need for bed rest because of this and the over-stretched abdominal muscles and pelvic ligaments. For the same reasons there is a greater need for physiotherapy to restore the body to normal and to prepare the woman for the extra load involved in caring for more than one baby. In this respect a visit from a member of the Multiple Birth Association while still in hospital can greatly assist the mother with advice and offers of help after she returns home.

POSTNATAL COMPLICATIONS

Although the postnatal phase is relatively uncomplicated in the vast majority of cases, there exists the possibility of some conditions which may be extremely serious: thrombosis of veins can lead to a blood clot which may become detached and lodge in the lungs; infection can occur in the genital organs and lead to blood poisoning; and other infections can occur in the breasts and in the urinary system. Finally, mental disturbances can develop which can have long-lasting results.

THROMBOSIS

Under normal conditions the blood inside the blood vessels remains fluid

A sore tummy
▼▼▼

One and one sometimes make four
▼▼▼

and does not clot. When a clot does form it is known as a thrombus and if this occurs in a vein it is called a venous thrombosis.

During pregnancy there are certain changes in the circulation which predispose to thrombus formation. The dilatation of the veins in the legs and the pelvis tends to slow down the flow of blood and changes occur in some constituents of the blood, both of which encourage clot formation. To some extent these changes are beneficial as they encourage the blood vessels exposed at the placental site to clot and to minimise the blood loss from the uterus after delivery.

However, if other factors such as uterine infection, prolonged bed rest and difficult labour are added, then clotting may occur in the dilated veins of the legs or of the pelvis. Should such a clot not be recognised it may leave the wall of the vein and lodge in the lungs where it produces a pulmonary embolus. This can be a serious and possibly a fatal condition.

Prevention is by leg exercises if confined to bed for any period of time during pregnancy, and by walking about soon after delivery. Early recognition of any red or tender areas in the calves or thighs which might indicate a thrombus allows treatment with an anti-coagulant to arrest and cure the condition.

POSTNATAL INFECTION

Infection occurring in the uterus after delivery, known as puerperal sepsis or by the older name of 'childbirth fever', was once a major cause of maternal death. Since the discovery of the sulphonamide drugs in 1936 and, later, penicillin, this condition has virtually disappeared. In addition, the improved management of obstetric complications, the increased safety of caesarean birth and the greater availability of blood transfusion have helped the maternal mortality rate dramatically improve from seven in every 1000 live births in 1936 to 30 in 100 000 between 1964–66 and then to 4 in 100 000 from 1985–87, which is the most recent data available at the moment.

Prevention of infection is still an important part of modern obstetric care and is one of the main reasons for recommending that all women be delivered in well-equipped obstetric units, staffed by highly trained midwives.

Early recognition of infection by regular recording of the temperature allows appropriate investigation and treatment to prevent any complication.

The lactating breast is another potential area for infection. The importance of correct care has been emphasised in Chapter 13: *What are my choices?*

Bladder and kidney infection can occur after childbirth if retention of urine is not recognised and treated.

MENTAL DISTURBANCES

While minor degrees of anxiety and depression are common following delivery, true psychotic illness is rare. However, both schizophrenia and depressive psychosis can recur or occur for the first time in the post-

Getting up early is important ▼▼▼

Postnatal infection – a rare complication ▼▼▼

partum period. If recognised early and treated correctly, the results are extremely good and, contrary to general belief, the condition does not always recur with subsequent pregnancies.

EMPTY HANDS

A few women may be without their babies in the labour and postnatal wards. This may be because the baby needs medical treatment and is in a special nursery or another hospital or, even more rarely, because the baby has died.

With the baby in a special nursery, not only is such a woman deprived of the gradual adjustment and 'getting to know you' process of the first few days but she also has the extra stress of worrying about her sick baby. A woman generally feels miserable and often blames herself for the baby's difficulties. Reassurance that she is blameless rarely stops her examining each detail of her pregnancy to try and find out what she did wrong. She may feel guilty and inadequate as a mother. Friends and relatives do not know what to say and many often avoid her or are overly cheerful, when she just feels like crying all the time. Being around other mothers happy with their babies is also distressing.

For such a woman the early visits to the baby can create great anxiety and she may feel a reluctance to see the child and get too close if she fears the child may not survive. Just as the mother of the healthy newborn has to adjust to the baby she has, rather than the ideal baby she has expected, so too does the mother of the special baby but for her there is an added intensity. In the same way, she has to accept her baby before she can really start to feel affection for the child.

Both parents share in these feelings of grief and need to live through them. There can be anger directed inwards at themselves or outwards at the doctors, hospital, God or just fate. There can be a degree of bargaining which takes the form of thoughts such as 'If only I do so and so, all will be well'. There will be depression and sadness but gradually, finally, will come the desire to face what has happened and make the best of it, and an ability to pick out all those good things in the baby despite the problems. At that point there can be planning for the future.

It is a lonely, empty feeling being in a ward without a baby, surrounded by other women busily caring for theirs, and having to visit the baby in the necessarily sterile surroundings of a special nursery. It is also very hard when it comes to leaving hospital without the baby and the feelings of disappointment and separation intensify.

Even though there are obstacles in the way of such a woman coming to know, care for and love her baby, she can do so. The process is a slow one and requires a lot of moral support from family and friends and constant visiting of the baby, helping in daily care and feeding when possible. Being able to provide baby with her own breast milk can give a real feeling of satisfaction.

Separation creates many problems
▼▼▼

Guilt
▼▼▼

Anger
▼▼▼

To enhance the couple's bonding to their baby in the special nursery, couples are able to visit any time of the day or night, older siblings are able to visit and a 'parents' room' has been established in most hospitals. Here parents can have a sleep or entertain older children or just 'have a break'. When the time comes for the baby to be discharged from the special nursery, mothers can 'board in' for several days. This enables new mothers who have missed out on caring for their child at birth because of his/her prematurity, to care for their baby full time before taking the baby home.

ABNORMALITIES

All couples fear the birth of a child with an abnormality. Such occurrences are relatively rare, but when an abnormality is evident, couples go through the same feelings of sadness and anger and disbelief mentioned above. This is a necessary step, and only after this are couples able to make the necessary plans for the ongoing care and welfare of their child. Some conditions are correctable e.g. cleft palates, whilst other problems require the couple to make special plans for the child's lifetime e.g. Down's Syndrome.

Whatever, it is extremely important that couples are advised about the supports and facilities available in the community, so that they do not go home feeling alone in the care of their baby. As such, visits are arranged for couples to meet self-help groups and Health Department professionals prior to discharge from the hospital. Such supports provide not only emotional help, but practical advice about caring for a special needs baby, and information about resources.

LOSING A BABY

In every 100 babies that are born, approximately one will die either soon after birth or be stillborn. In either case it is a tragic and crushing blow to the parents. Even though they have hardly seen their baby, he or she is a member of the family and the parents grieve for the loss deeply. Their knowledge of the baby is confined to perhaps a short time after birth, and to the kicks and movements while in the womb but after the baby is gone there are so few tangible memories to compensate for the intense pain of separation. Photos of the baby may assist to make the situation more real, but no less painful.

In a vain attempt to cushion the blow, our mind tends to play tricks on us. Firstly, it tries to get us to deny that the problem exists e.g. 'I just can't believe it', 'I still feel pregnant', and almost a feeling that this is happening to somebody else. Unfortunately this doesn't help for long and is one of the reasons why it is so important that parents see and hold their baby, during and after death. It gives parents the chance to say goodbye, to feel involved, and to have some close physical contact, however short-lived, with their baby. With every mother and father there is a 'cuddle that must come out' which if left inside can cause the pain of separation to be greater. The mind becomes 'numb' in an attempt to deal with the situation and this also increases the sense of unreality.

Such is the enormity of the tragedy that a couple may experience a sense of complete calm — at least for a short while.

Soon, however, these feelings give way to severe suffering and depression. This can be so intense as to cause real physical pain. At the same time, a lot of anger may be felt. This may be directed outwards to the hospital, the doctors or nurses, or even 'fate' or 'God', or directed inward creating feelings of intense guilt. Both the mother and father may experience mood swings, sometimes feeling in control and at other times bottomless heartache. This is the nature of grieving: the 'pangs' that come and go for weeks and months after the loss.

Despite the sadness, anger and other feelings associated with the loss of the baby, there are decisions that have to be made at this time and generally these should be made while still in hospital. Specifically, the birth of the child must be registered. This is a requirement for any child born over 20 weeks gestation and applies even to the stillborn child. Decisions have to be made about burial and cremation of the baby, whether or not a service with the family and friends in attendance is desired and so on. Whatever, it is very important that the couple whose baby has died are involved in the decision making. This may be painful at the time, but it is an essential part of the grieving process.

As the numbness wears off, the pangs usually get worse and the pain increases. Often several weeks after the baby dies instead of coping better the couple may still be unable to bear the grief. This adjustment may take months or years. In some cases it may even be delayed. By refusing to see or hold the baby at birth, by rushing around and pretending that nothing has happened, by getting back to work as quickly as possible, maintaining a façade of 'coping well', or by taking tranquillisers or other drugs, the feelings of pain are suppressed. This does not make the feelings any less painful. Instead they begin to affect other parts of life and other relationships and eventually they will have to be faced. It is only by going through and dealing with the depression and emptiness, that it can be integrated into the routine of daily life, finally allowing life to move ahead.

After several months, or sometimes after a year, the memories of the baby lose their pain but the sadness remains. When this occurs it is, perhaps, time to consider another pregnancy. The new baby will then be a person in his or her own right and not a replacement baby for the one just lost.

It is a difficult time for the relationship between the father and the mother. Relationships can be made worse or better by such crises. Worse, if in order to protect each other, the partners stop talking about their grief. But better if the couple grow closer through their mutual pain with open communication and understanding.

Parents often say that losing a baby teaches them compassion for others and to appreciate the things that they have, and the wonder of a healthy baby is not in any way lost by their experience, however difficult to bear.

'The cuddle that must come out'
▼▼▼

Difficult decisions have to be made
▼▼▼

Another baby
▼▼▼

CHAPTER 15

I DIDN'T KNOW IT WOULD BE LIKE THIS

Going Home

For some families a new baby is a total joy, with no unexpected stresses and no impossible situations. Unfortunately, this is not always the case.

Packing up in anticipation of leaving hospital sometimes gives a little insight into the next few months. Between feeding and bathing the baby, then showering and dressing in clothes that do not fit, the effort of going home can be quite an ordeal. Most women want to get away from the fixed hospital routine but many are aware that readily available help will be scarce at home.

Packing up can be a business

▼▼▼

The hospital bill is paid, the goodbyes and the thankyous said. Then, at most hospitals, a nurse actually puts the baby in the mother's arms at the front door. In a way this symbolises the transfer of responsibility from hospital to parent.

TIME *to* GO

Going home with a new baby is a special and happy time. Although a mother faces the responsibility and even the fear of being totally in charge of her baby's care, she may also for the first time really feel the baby is hers and is not shared with anyone else but her partner. For the father this is also a special time. Proud of his partner and new child he is also acutely aware of their possible dependence on him. This can be worrying and if he feels he has lost some of his partner's attention and loving to the new baby, he can feel resentful, lonely and unable to share his feelings.

By the time they go home, that special bond between mother and child is well on its way to being cemented. However, it is now time for new bonds to be developed between father and child and it takes all members of the family to participate in developing the changed relationship that will lead to a workable future.

AT HOME

New parents tend to go and look at the baby every few minutes when they first get home. Fortunately, this need to see if he or she is still beautiful passes fairly quickly. If the need is to see if the baby is still breathing, then this is an expression of anxiety. For some parents it will pass as they realise that babies are not fragile; for others this anxiety may increase and ruin the enjoyment they should get from their baby.

SOCIAL PRESSURES ON PARENTS

There are many social and community attitudes and pressures which make parenthood more rather than less difficult. The most important of these may be the denigration of mothering as a full-time, worthwhile occupation. Women who see mothering as a useful profession manage it very much better than those who remain in conflict between their previous occupation and their role as mothers.

It is an advantage if, early on, both partners work out their respective parental roles as best they can before reality hits home. It follows that their respective community roles will be settled also. Women who return to work soon after the baby's birth must delegate the mothering role satisfactorily to avoid tremendous guilt feelings.

There is a social pressure on some parents not to change their lifestyle just for the baby: 'The baby must fit in with us.' Many problems arise when new parents persist with this view despite its obvious absurdity. How can a three member unit be the same as a two member unit? Families who cannot accept a baby's basic demands for food and loving, which includes close contact and time, must have difficulties.

The pressure to succeed in parenthood is a social pressure as well as an individual one. It may seem that everyone to whom new parents talk had no problems and had perfect babies who slept all night from the moment they got home from hospital. Most of these people have forgotten, or are making it up, or are refusing to admit their own failures. Few offer help, most criticise and create a feeling of incompetence and failure.

Mothering is an occupation too
▼▼▼

You usually fit in with baby
▼▼▼

*You are
going to feel
tired*
▼▼▼

*... so don't
make it worse
than it is*
▼▼▼

*The pressure
can come
from yourself*
▼▼▼

*Or from
other people*
▼▼▼

PHYSICAL PRESSURES ON PARENTS

A baby who wakes for feeds every three and a half to four hours through the night does not allow for long periods of sleep, unless the partner can give a bottle (which is unwise for the breastfed baby in the early months). Even if the mother goes to bed soon after the evening meal, the lack of a significant period of sleep at night creates fatigue and its associated problems. This can go on for about six weeks until the baby no longer needs one of the night feeds. The fatigue is often increased by the extra load of washing, the extra load of afternoon teas for the inevitable and perhaps inconsiderate visitors and possibly left-over tiredness from the actual labour and delivery.

Occasionally some women load themselves with unnecessary physical work by preparing special meals for guests, moving house, preparing the nursery, or commencing some outside job within weeks of getting home.

Needless to say, the workload with twins is more than doubled but hopefully women manage because they have two arms and a strong will. With triplets, outside help is probably essential. Joining organisations like the Multiple Birth Association is very worthwhile as all the members know just what is involved.

Early on, new mothers must try to organise a daytime sleep for themselves. It is very easy if there is only one child and is not impossible if the other is under three years of age. If there are two children in the house when the third arrives, a day sleep may be impossible without extra help.

SELF-IMPOSED PRESSURES

Many mothers put themselves under extreme pressure to prove that they are perfect mothers, perfect partners, perfect housekeepers, all at once. This desire is often totally unrealistic when a young mother comes home with her first baby.

One of the first lessons for the new mother is to give all activities a priority rating and not to get uptight if some things are not done for days and days and days. It is usually impossible for mothers to do everything they have planned in any given day. The house-proud woman who likes her home to be immaculate may feel especially unhappy with this new situation.

If this pressure to be 'perfect' is coming from the father, he should be given an evening alone with the baby to see what it is really like. If it is coming from relatives or friends, they must be dealt with promptly before they disturb the new family. No matter how perfect they may seem to be as parents, nobody must be allowed to dictate to the new mother and father.

One of the most pressing problems early on is the realisation that time alone to do what one wants and to think one's own thoughts is almost impossible to obtain. If the need for this is great, it may be necessary to get a babysitter early. This might be father, grandmother, a neighbour or a friend. If none of these are immediately available, ask the local baby clinic sister to find a suitable person nearby. Swapping baby-minding time with other mothers is the easiest way to get time off.

This loss of individual freedom is often one of the hardest parts of the new lifestyle of the three unit family. When a woman has trouble accepting this loss, she is likely to remain tense, angry and guilty. Her baby will not relax, will sleep poorly, will cry excessively and will be diagnosed as having colic. A father is less aware of the problems if he has a full-time job and is not at home for long periods of time.

EMOTIONAL PRESSURES ON THE MOTHER

Women are often 'emotional' for some time after leaving hospital. This is due to a combination of factors, such as physical tiredness, continual worry about the baby and problems related to the role of mother.

Most parents worry about their children. Guilt feelings are also very common in the early period. Uncertainties about what is the right thing to do leave a mother open to guilt feelings whichever way she goes. A lot of these are a hangover from what she believes were her inadequacies at the time of delivery.

One of the greatest emotional pressures on the mother is the realisation that her baby is totally dependent on her. Some mothers love this feeling but some are almost terrified by it. Occasionally a mother is so obsessive about her baby that she will not let anyone else handle, feed, bath or babysit her baby. This may be an expression of extreme anxiety and should be discussed with the baby clinic sister or other professionals.

EMOTIONAL PRESSURES ON THE FATHER

The traditional view of the Australian male has been that he is supposed to be uninterested in babies, does not want to help and is more involved with 'the boys' than with home life. If the father is like that and will not change, he will be a problem! If he wants to change these attitudes, then he must be helped to do so. The involvement of fathers is now the more accepted approach.

Fathers must know how much physical and emotional strain is involved in child-rearing. They should learn to help physically with meals, housekeeping, shopping and so on. They should help emotionally with making decisions, and by telling his partner how well she is coping, as too few people are likely to be supportive.

The father will quickly realise that communication with his partner is very difficult early on when she is tired, unstable and worried. Accordingly, he should be considerate and understanding, particularly in the re-establishment of sexual relationships.

He cannot afford to be the anxious one in the house. His role is to ease the load, not to add to the pressures. If he has to be away for any length of time, he should be aware of the increased emotional load this adds to his partner.

Fathers soon realise that the baby's responses to him are different from those received by the mother. Mothers are often a testing ground for new skills whereas father is a play object. However with increased

Most parents worry
▼▼▼

Fathers can do more
▼▼▼

'sharing of the load' this role division does not necessarily occur. These different responses do not represent more love or more caring by the child for the father — it is just that the child may have and continue to always have a different relationship with the mother and the father.

EMOTIONAL PRESSURES ON OTHER CHILDREN

All children may see a new baby as a challenge to their being loved and to their importance. However, in the early weeks at home, children under three are likely still to be angry with mother for having left them to go to hospital. Children's anger is directed against her, irrespective of how well they have been looked after during her absence. When she comes home, under-three year olds may seek attention by misbehaving and clinging. Neither of these activities help the tired mother, but the children's basic need is there and must be answered. Children will only get jealous of the new baby if they are pushed away at feed time or bath time or not allowed contact with the baby. Children can sit next to mother at feed time and be talked or read to. They will ask only once for a taste of the breast milk, because they will not like it. They can help with bathing and play time. Of course, they must be taught the adult way of holding cuddling, stroking or playing with babies.

BABIES' DEMANDS

Many women are taken totally by surprise by their babies when they get home. They may not have expected the forcefulness with which babies make their presence felt. Few babies can be ignored if they want to be noticed.

Mothers seem to expect babies to wake often and feed often. They are sometimes surprised by the baby's need for cuddling and contact time. The need is individual; some babies get their full quota at feed time and some need much more. Some may only want it at particular times of the day and some mothers are upset by the fact that it is usually at the least convenient time.

Babies object violently to being bustled. They like a quiet, peaceful, easy life. Any attempts to hurry the feed, rush baby off to sleep, whip clothes on and off, will lead to loud objections. And why shouldn't baby object?

In the first couple of months babies need to relax after feeds in order to go to sleep. Some need this desperately! Babies cannot relax unless the mother is relaxed. This interchange of emotional tension between mother (and father) and child is very strong but some mothers cannot always see it. There are many days when mother knows she is uptight from the time she gets up — she knows she will have a bad day — and then the baby plays up. There are also bad days which begin with baby in a bad mood for a host of possible reasons.

There are truly difficult babies but these should be checked out medically for a number of possible diseases. After that, there are still some babies and infants who are hard to live with for reasons that may never be found.

BABIES' BEHAVIOUR

Parents spend a great deal of time worrying about the natural activities of their baby. This applies especially to eating and sleeping.

Feeding is a totally natural activity and, when food is available, feeding is easy and automatically successful. It does not have to be taught or learned. However, parents tend to interfere excessively with their baby's appetites. If babies are hungry, they scream; if they do not get enough food at a feeding, they look around for more; if they get too much milk, they might bring it up. Like their parents they do not like to drink the same amount at every feed or be fed at exactly the same time every day, or be given food they do not like.

In the first three to four months, most babies are happy to drink only milk with occasional drinks of water or orange juice. Feeding may be quite irregular in the early weeks, but later a three to four hourly schedule usually develops until three meals a day are indicated. One night feed usually drops out in the second month of life. The other night feed may take a further four to six months to go. These drop away naturally without training.

The need for sleep naturally follows a feeling of tiredness and this occurs frequently in babies. A few minutes of laughter or of being passed around to several adults, all of whom want to 'goo' and 'gaa' can be hard work for a small baby. Whenever babies (in the first four months at least) are tired, as shown by yawning, drooping eyelids and particularly by crying, they should be allowed to sleep. Over-excitement can interfere with the relaxation necessary for a tired baby to drop off to sleep. In such cases it is not the tiredness or the desire to sleep which is unnatural, it is the over-excitement.

SUPPORT SYSTEMS

It is necessary for most mothers to have one or two people who can help her physically and emotionally with child rearing. These may be her own mother, or mother-in-law, relatives or friends.

It is common to get little physical help and vast amounts of verbal advice, much of which is inappropriate, conflicting, or frankly unreasonable. Unfortunately, the inexperienced mother may listen to it all, try to incorporate all of it into her daily routine and gets more and more confused.

Mothers do have natural instincts which tell them what is right for their baby. These may be hidden behind over-intellectualisation or smothered by anxiety, but they are there and should be used.

Before you are discharged from hospital you will be given details of the services of your local Baby Health Centre which will be able to offer you support, encouragement and practical advice. Contact with other community services which may be considered to be of assistance can also be arranged.

RELAXATION

Relaxation continues to be of prime importance to the mother. The need to relax will be felt many times during

Nature knows best
▼▼▼

Never hesitate to ask for help
▼▼▼

the day for perhaps short periods of time. Get into the habit of being able to sign off from situations, concentrating on easy breathing, consciously letting tension dissipate. Hopefully this may almost become a habit. Use relaxation to try to promote sleep even for short spells. It may even improve the quality of sleep. Something that all new mothers need to realise is that long periods of sleep are impossible for the time being. New fathers are not exempt from this situation either, so they can also benefit from relaxation.

EXERCISE

The simple prenatal exercises for the muscles around the breasts may be continued and again thought should be given to the correct support for the breasts as lactation increases. The question of girdles sometimes arises, though not so often since the advent of pantihose. If the need to wear one occurs, there is no harm whatsoever, as long as the girdle is not expected to do all the work. It should be remembered that nature has provided a built-in support in the abdominal muscles and first thoughts should be to maintain these muscles in good tone. Separation of the long, straight muscles in the mid-line of the abdomen occurs to many women in pregnancy and persists postnatally; some mothers find that extra support is needed until these muscles regain full strength.

Having left the comparative security of the hospital, the home exercise programme needs to be considered. Time is everyone's enemy but perhaps even more so for new mothers. There is probably little or no

time for the organised exercise programme of the hospital. If there is such time, try to arrange it for the morning and use the afternoon for relaxation. Better still, try to incorporate exercise in the form of body awareness into as many ordinary activities of daily living as possible. Place a mark of some kind in the parts of the house most used: the bathroom mirror, the laundry, kitchen sink, refrigerator, clothes hoist and the pram to name a few. Each time you see a mark it will remind you to check muscle function and posture.

Lifting is an activity that must be performed most carefully at all times. The correct method is to bend the knees, keeping the back straight and carrying the load as close to the body as possible. This ensures that the back muscles and ligaments are not put under any undue strain. Also, put objects to be lifted in places where bending is reduced, for example, a washing basket on a surface at waist-level before filling it. And remember that dividing a load will help.

Progress can be made without your realising it. Days since delivery become weeks and then months. There is no exact moment when involution is complete and muscles and ligaments return to normal, so there is no cut-off point for doing exercises. Hopefully the programme of postnatal exercises will become a comfortable habit, with benefit to both mother and baby.

MENSTRUAL PERIODS

By six weeks, a menstrual period may have occurred in the woman who is bottle feeding.

The interval before menstruation returns and the character of the period vary enormously. Some women get no periods for months, especially when breastfeeding and even more especially if they are using a progesterone-only oral contraceptive pill. One of the real blessings of pregnancy is that heavy or painful periods are often cured after childbirth. Nobody can predict when periods will return; it is a case of wait and see.

SEX

The age-old excuse of 'Not tonight, I'm too tired' must surely have been said by many a new mother. It is not due to a lack of love; indeed, the woman is highly dependent upon her partner at this difficult time. It is a combination of many things. The first and most important is the draining of mental energy which makes 'turning on' difficult. Some men may welcome this time not to be expected to perform. Others, however, may complain, placing an unfair additional strain on the woman. He will manage despite his grumbling.

Another important reason is the natural fear of falling pregnant too soon, which switches off any amorous desires. It takes anything up to six months, though usually not that long, for sufficient physical and emotional reserves to have been recovered to cope with the possibility of another baby. Fortunately modern contraception does away with much of this fear, but the natural fear lingers anyway.

The low level of oestrogen is another reason for not feeling particularly sexually adventurous at this time. The best way to test this personally is to note the dryness and lack of secretions in the vaginal skin when sexual activity is attempted. Obviously the scar tissue from stitches or a small tear will cause the vaginal opening to be less flexible and even a little sore. For most people it takes love, understanding and possibly a lubricant to get things working properly after a baby. Despite this, after several attempts most people find that the vagina is beginning to get more supple and moist.

It is a time for giving love and for understanding each other. Hopefully neither you nor your partner will be too embarrassed to talk about any difficulties. Sexual problems after childbirth are becoming less common nowadays but they do still occur and, if allowed to persist, can lead to a chronic breakdown of the relationship.

CONTRACEPTION

The techniques available are the same as before you had the baby, but the application of these techniques may not be appropriate until periods are regular again, or the womb is back to ordinary size, or breastfeeding has stopped.

It is important to talk about contraception with the obstetrician before leaving hospital. Another baby before the first birthday of the previous one represents an enormous physical burden, if nothing else.

The woman who is not breastfeeding can ovulate as early as one month after childbirth and fall pregnant again. She needs contraceptive advice before leaving

The resumption of sexual activity should be a mutual decision
▼▼▼

hospital and the choices open to her partner are abstinence, or the use of condoms. She can commence an oral contraceptive pill but cannot usually be fitted with a diaphragm or an intra-uterine device until the sixth week when the uterus and vagina have returned to a normal size. Following her first menstrual period she can use the ovulation method, combining observation of the cervical mucus with daily temperature recordings.

On the other hand, women who are fully breastfeeding will not ovulate for at least two months, and many of them will be protected for six months or more. Less than 2 per cent of women conceive before the sixth month after childbirth and some neither ovulate nor menstruate while they continue to lactate, even when they are not fully breastfeeding. The ordinary oral contraceptive pill is not advisable as the oestrogen in it inevitably suppresses milk production. However, a progesterone-only pill may be ordered which does not interfere with lactation. All the other methods of birth control are also applicable after the second month but some women choose to avoid contraception and allow another pregnancy to occur. This is the case when another child is wanted fifteen to twenty months later, or if there has been a worrying phase of infertility before the first child was conceived.

However, when it is important for personal reasons to avoid another pregnancy for two to three years, it would be most unwise to rely on the protection given by breastfeeding. In these cases a more effective contraceptive technique should be chosen from the available range.

POSTNATAL EXAMINATION

In most cases the uterus will have returned to its normal size, (though it will always be slightly larger than before the pregnancy), some six weeks after delivery. So it is no coincidence that this is the time usually suggested for the postnatal examination. It is a convenient time to check the progress of the mother and baby and to plan for the future. On the other hand the request made to the mother on leaving hospital that the obstetrician wishes to see her when the baby is six weeks old is sometimes construed as disinterest in what happens over the next four to five weeks. This is not so, and parents are encouraged to maintain contact and seek advice for any problem.

The examination itself is usually a happy and relaxed affair with mother and baby showing how well they have learned to cope with each other. Problems that may have occurred during the pregnancy and labour are discussed again and their possible significance for future pregnancies is talked over. There is an opportunity to examine the baby, although this role is being taken over increasingly by the paediatrician who saw the baby in hospital.

It is wise for the father to be present also, so that both parents can discuss with the doctor the effect of the new baby on the family. In addition, the presence of other children allows the doctor to assess how they are coping with the new arrival.

The examination of the woman is concerned mainly with the return to normal of the uterus and vagina. A cancer detection smear is usually taken during the pelvic examination and routine tests of urine and blood pressure are performed. The mother's weight should be no more than 2 to 3 kg above her pre-pregnancy weight, but she may still be concerned about her flabby abdomen. This is a good time to emphasise the need for post-natal exercises (see pages 176) which tend to be forgotten in the busy few weeks after returning home. There is still a need for regular rest periods and the father's assistance can be very valuable at this time.

Where a caesarean birth was necessary, the wound is carefully examined. The scar is usually red and often itchy, both of which problems will fade over the next few months. When the scar is across the lower abdomen there is often numbness along the top of the scar and a deeper ridge of thickening beneath it. The numbness disappears in another month as the tiny nerves that have been cut slowly regenerate. The ridge of tissue is caused by stitches in the deeper layers of the abdominal wall and can be expected to shrink and disappear by the third month. It is usually possible to predict whether a normal or a caesarean birth will be necessary in a subsequent pregnancy.

Contraceptive techniques are the other important items for discussion and the parents should take the opportunity to talk about the resumption of sexual activity.

A pat on the back and a word of praise are important ingredients and the consultation ends with congratulations all round.

Mother and baby both need to be examined

▼ ▼ ▼

CONCLUSION

A new baby can make physical demands on the mother that are much greater than expected. The emotional demands, and the way they are met, depend on the personalities, the hopes and the aspirations of the parents and their knowledge and experience of children.

If parents can appreciate that babies are not possessions to be managed and manipulated, but people with needs and desires to be met, then the rearing of children can be the most rewarding of all life's experiences.

GLOSSARY

Anencephaly Defective development of the brain, together with absence of the bones of the cranial vault.

Anterior In front of; in the front part of.

Cystic fibrosis An inherited disorder affecting the pancreas, lungs and sweat glands.

Embryo The baby in its first 12 weeks of development in the uterus.

Fetus The baby from the 12th week of its development until delivery.

Fundus The uppermost point of the pregnant uterus.

Gestation Period of time between conception and birth.

Haemophilia An inherited disorder of the blood: a permanent tendency towards haemorrhages due to a defect in the coagulating power of the blood.

Lateral On the side of; further from the median.

Low birthweight Less than 2500 grams.

Multigravida A woman who has been pregnant two or more times previously.

Multipara A woman who has been delivered of two or more children with gestational ages of 20 weeks or more, irrespective of whether or not they were born alive.

Muscular dystrophy This describes a group of inherited diseases characterised by weakness in muscles and associated wasting of certain muscle groups.

Post-term After 42 weeks.

Posterior Behind; at the back of.

Pre-term Before 37 weeks.

Premature This is an old term which was much used and confused in obstetrics in referring to babies, labour and so on. More accurate World Health Organisation definitions are now available, so the term has been dropped, apart from its use referring to rupture of the membranes before the onset of labour.

Primigravida A woman who is pregnant for the first time.

Primipara A woman who has been delivered of an infant with a gestational age of 20 weeks or more, irrespective of whether the infant was alive or not.

Puerperium The period from the end of labour to complete involution (shrinkage) of the uterus. There is no exact time definition for puerperium.

Spina bifida A congenital defect of the spine which allows the spinal membranes (with or without spinal cord tissue) to protrude.

Term Between 38 and 42 weeks.

Thalassaemia An inherited disorder found particularly in individuals living in countries bordering in the Mediterranean. It is characterised by the presence of unusually thin red blood cells and varying degrees of anaemia.

INDEX

complexion, mother's 42
confidence 160
congenital abnormalities *see* abnormalities
constipation, baby's 142
constipation, mother's 43
contraception 177-8
contractions
  Braxton-Hicks 43, 73, 99
  breathing 69
  during pregnancy 73
  induction 104
  monitoring 111
  onset of labour 100-1
  first stage of labour 106, 108
  second stage of labour 122
controlled breathing 68-9
convenience foods 65
corpus luteum 11
costal breathing 68-9
courtesy card 58
cramps
  abdominal 25
  during pregnancy 44
CVS 23, 97
cystic fibrosis 23, 96

dating the embryo 21-2
deformities *see* abnormalities
delivery 120-31
  breech 130
  events following 126-8
  Leboyer method 127
  placenta and membranes 131
  second stage of labour 123-6
depression, postnatal 159-60
descent of the baby 109-10
diabetes 52, 53, 91-2, 93-4
diagnostic ultrasound 97
diaphragm 78
diet during pregnancy 38, 40, 43
digestive tract, baby's 83
dilatation of the cervix 99, 109
diseases during pregnancy 59, 93-4
dislocation of the hip 144
disproportion 112-13
  caesarean section 135
dizzy spells 40
doctor
  prenatal visits 51-3, 57-8
  when and which to see 50
Down's Syndrome 22-3, 96
dreams 32-3
drugs
  medicinal *see* medication
  recreational 22, 59

early childhood centres 65
ears, baby's 84
eating
  see also nutrition
  during labour 109
eclampsia 89
ectoderm 17, 19
ectopic pregnancy 26
EDD 37-8, 102
education 65-9, 114-15
egg cell 15, 16
embryo
  see also fetus
  fertilisation 12
  growth 13-21, 81
  measuring 80
embryology 21
embryonic disc 17-18
emotions
  during pregnancy 28-35
  after delivery 158-9
  after leaving hospital 173
endoderm 17, 18
engagement of the head 71, 110
epidural anaesthesia
  caesarean section 136, 137
  forceps delivery 130
  normal delivery 117-18
epidural catheter 117
epilepsy 94
episiotomy 128, 164
epistaxis 48
estimated date of delivery 37-8, 102
examination of baby 138-51, 144, 178-9
examination of mother during pregnancy 53
exercises
  during pregnancy 58, 66-7
  for labour 115
  postnatal 163, 165, 176-7
expectations 157
expected date of delivery 37-8, 102
eyes, baby's
  fetus 85
  examination 139
  sticky 145-6
eyes, mother's, during pregnancy 45

face, baby's 84, 85
fainting 40
faintness 68
Fallopian tubes 26
false labour 101
family history 52
fantasies 32-3
fat necrosis 145

fathers
  after birth 171
  anxiety 34
  emotional pressures 173-4
  fatherhood 29
  postnatal examinations 178
fatigue
  during pregnancy 39
  after birth 172
  early pregnancy 30
FBS 97
fear of pregnancy 177
feeding 148-53, 175
fertilisation 11-12
  cell division 15
  division of the egg 16
fertility 9-10
fetal blood sampling 97
fetus
  see also baby; embryo
  abnormalities *see* abnormalities
  amniotic fluid 76
  blood supply 74-5
  delivery 123-6
  descent 109-10
  distress 111-12, 129, 130, 135
  effect on mother 71
  growth and development 21-2, 80-7
  kicking 42
  measurement 80, 95
  miscarriage 24-6
  monitoring during labour 111-12
  movement 84, 86
  tests 95-8
finger nails, baby's 147
fits during pregnancy 89
fluid retention 46
fontanelle 87, 139
food *see* nutrition
forceps delivery 129-30
  aftereffects 164-5
foreskins 155
fruit 63

gazing reflex 127
genes 14-15
genetic defects 23-3, 96-7
genitals, baby's 140
German measles 22, 54
gestation table 37
glucometer 93
granuloma 143
grasp reflex 141
grief
  abnormalities 168
  absent baby 167

Group B Streptococcus
  screening 56
growth retardation 57, 91-2
guilt 173
gums, mother's, during pregnancy 45

haemoglobin, baby's 143
haemoglobin, mother's 53
haemophilia 23
haemorrhoids 43, 44
hair, baby's
  fetus 84, 87
  examination 139
hair, mother's, growth during pregnancy 42
hands, mother's, painful 48
harness 144
hCG 26-7, 36
head, baby's
  fetus 85, 87
  during birth 110
  examination 139
  shape 141-2
headaches 47
heart, baby's
  development 20
  abnormalities 22
  growth 81
  fetus 85
  during labour 111, 112
  after delivery 126
heart, mother's
  disease 94
  during pregnancy 77
heartburn 45-6
height, mother's 53
hernias in baby 140
heroin 59
high blood pressure *see* hypertension
hips, baby's
  clicky 144-5
  examination 140
HIV testing 56
home after birth 170-9
hormones 10-11
  breastfeeding 149
  during pregnancy 84
  mood changes 31
hospitals
  admission 102-3, 105
  labour preparation classes 66
  leaving 99-105, 170-1
  place to have baby 50
  rooming-in 153
house moving 34
HPL 96
human chorionic gonadotrophin 26-7, 36

posture, mother's
    during pregnancy 67, 78, 79
    after delivery 164
pre-eclampsia *see* hypertension
pre-eclamptic toxaemia *see*
    hypertension
pre-term labour 92, 103
    caesarean section 134
    forceps 130
    multiple pregnancies 90
    prenatal visits 57
preparation for pregnancy 7-12
presenting part 99
problem pregnancies 88-98
progesterone 11, 78
prostaglandins 60, 104
psychoprophylaxis 114-16
psychosis 166
pudendal block 118
pyridoxine 38

quadruplets 27
quickening 84

Read, Dr Grantly Dick 114
recreational drugs cause of
    abnormalities 22, 59
red blood cells 77
reduction division 15
reflexes 140-1
relatives 158
relaxation
    after birth 175-6
    baby 153
    exercises 69, 115
rest during pregnancy 59
resuscitation 126
Rhesus iso-immunisation 25,
    53, 75, 94-5
ribs, mother's 47, 78
Ritodrine 92
rooming-in 153-4
Royal Hospital for Women,
    Paddington, NSW 49, 153
rubella 22, 54

sciatica 48
sex chromosomes 14
sex determination 15-16
sexual activity
    during pregnancy 32, 60
    after birth 176-7
show 101
shower 162
sitting
    during pregnancy 68
    during labour 122
skeleton, baby's 83
skeleton, mother's 78

skin, baby's
    fetus 84, 85, 86
    after delivery 139
skin, mother's
    changes during pregnancy
        42
    during pregnancy 78
    itching 45
    stretch marks 41
sleep, baby 175
sleeplessness, mother, during
    pregnancy 46-7
smoking 22, 52, 163
snacks 63
sneezes 145
Snow, John 113
snuffles 145
social pressures on parents 171
somites 20, 81
sperm cells 11, 15
spider naevi 78
spina bifida 54, 61, 96
spinal column development 20-1
spontaneous abortion 24-6, 93
squatting position for labour 122
standing
    during pregnancy 67
    during delivery 121
    after delivery 164
startle reflex 140-1
sticky eyes 145
stillborn 168
stirrups 130
stitches 164
stork bites 139
strawberry marks 139
Streptococcus 56
stress incontinence 128
stretch marks 41
striae 41
support stockings 44
surfactant 92
swallowing movements, baby's
    83
synctocinon 104, 112, 133
syntometrine 131
syphilis 54

take-away foods 65
tears
    during pregnancy 31
    after delivery 160
teenagers 64
teeth, mother's, during
    pregnancy 45
temperature, baby's 142
termination of pregnancy 24
testosterone 11

tests
    fetus 95-8
    for abnormalities 23-4
    for pregnancy 36-7
    mother 53-7
tetracyclines 59
thalassaemia 96
thalidomide 22
thrombosis 165-6
thrush 45
tiredness *see* fatigue
tobacco 22, 52, 163
toxic erythema 145
transition 108
translocation 25
travel during pregnancy 60
trial of labour 104-5
triplets 27
trophoblast 18
trophoblastic cells 17, 18, 74
tumours 27, 135
twins 90-1
    delivery 119
    development 80
    diagnosis 96
    family history 52
    fertilisation 27
    labour 130-1
    workload 172

ultrasound 56-7, 95-6
    how it works 81
    hydatidiform mole 27
    measuring the embryo 80
    monitoring labour 111
    testing for abnormalities 24
umbilical cord 140, 142-3
    clamping 126
    description 75
    growth 18
unexpected pregnancies 34
uniovular twins 27, 90
unplanned pregnancy 9
upper uterine segment 100
urine, baby's 142
urine, mother's
    after delivery 162
    during pregnancy 39
    incontinence 46
    sample 57
    test 37, 53
uterus
    after delivery 131-2, 133
    blood supply 73-4
    contractions *see* contractions
    during implantation 17
    during pregnancy 71-2, 78
    early stages of pregnancy 18
    enlargement 41

muscles 100
    postnatal examination 179
    shrinking 161
    size 57

vagina
    bleeding *see* vaginal
        bleeding
    discharge during
        pregnancy 40
    during delivery 123-4
    during pregnancy 74
    examination 58
    laceration 133
    postnatal examination 179
    secretions 74
    tears 128
vaginal bleeding
    baby 147
    early pregnancy 26-7
    miscarriage 25
Valium 44
varicose veins 44, 74, 78
VDRL 54
vegetarians 65
veɪ.ous thrombosis 166
Ventolin 92
ventouse suction cup 129
vernix caseosa 85, 87
version 86
viability 85
vitamin B6 38
vomiting
    baby 146
    mother 30, 31, 38
vulva 74

walking reflex 141
waters, breaking of 75-65, 101
weight, baby's 152
weight, mother's
    gain after delivery 163
    gain during pregnancy 40,
        63-4, 79-80
    measurement 53, 57
    multiple pregnancy 80
womb
    body *see* uterus
    neck *see* cervix
working during pregnancy,
    39, 58-9

X chromosomes 14
X-linked abnormalities 23
X-ray examination of pelvis 91

Y chromosomes 14
yolk sac 17